Handprints

Home Programs for Hand Skills

by
Valerie Pieraccini, OTR/L
and
Darla K. Vance, M.S., OTR/L

Foreword by Marsha Dunn Klein, M.Ed., OTR/L

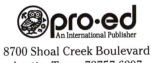

8700 Shoal Creek Boulevard
Austin, Texas 78757-6897
800/897-3202   Fax 800/397-7633
www.proedinc.com

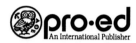

© 2001 by PRO-ED, Inc.
8700 Shoal Creek Boulevard
Austin, Texas 78757-6897
800/897-3202   Fax 800/397-7633
www.proedinc.com

Edited by Nancy Weaver and Jody Cosson

Illustrations by Christine McNamara

Cover by Deborah Nore

Library of Congress Cataloging-in-Publication Data

Pieraccini, Valerie, 1964-
    Handprints : home programs for hand skills / by Valerie Pieraccini, and Darla K. Vance.
        p.cm.
    Includes bibliographical references.
    ISBN 1-883315-56-5
    1. Movement disorders in children—Treatment—Handbooks, manuals, etc. 2. Motor
ability in children—Handbooks, manuals, etc. 3. Handicapped
children—Education—Handbooks, manuals, etc. 4. Occupational therapy for
children—Handbooks, manuals, etc. I. Vance, Darla K., 1996- II. Title.

RJ496.M68 P53 2001
618.92'7—dc21

                                                                    2001024155

Printed in the United States of America

    2   3   4   5   6   7   8   9   10   08   07   06   05   04

Dedication

To my mother, Ann Curley, who encouraged me to become an occupational therapist—I'm so glad I followed her advice.

Valerie Pieraccini

To my family, for giving me enough enthusiastic support, encouragement and humor for a lifetime.

Darla K. Vance

Acknowledgments

When you work on a project of this magnitude, there are always many people who should be thanked. We have people who have helped us as individuals and those who have helped us jointly.

I, Valerie, want to thank the following: The Lord Jesus Christ for His faithfulness to me throughout all of life. My husband, Paul Pieraccini, for the way he loves and cares for me. Neither I nor my computer would have made it through this project without him. My parents, Virgil and Ann Curley, whose constant support—whether with school, babies or books—has allowed me to do all that I have done. Darla Vance, who I hardly knew when we entered into this project but who has been a great partner and friend. Her patience has been amazing with the constant commotion in my house. Jayme Johnston, whose help with my house and children allowed me to give birth to a book and a baby all in one summer. My children, Lucas and Alex, whose hand skills unfolded even as I wrote this book—and who gave me inspiration to write.

I, Darla, want to thank the following: My Dad, L. Jon Schurmeier, who taught me that I could do anything I set my mind to. My Mom, Donna Kay Cunningham, who has always been there. My sisters, Kristin Wallace and Steff Toppin, for being my best friends. Monty Vance, for his love and for having confidence in me. Valerie Pieraccini, for inviting me into this project and being a true friend through a vast amount of writes, rewrites, e-mails, and discussions. The incredible mentors and teachers I have been fortunate enough to learn from in my years as a therapist: Nancy Bagatell, Bonnie Boenig, Judy Calgagno, Kathy Deverna and Marsha Dunn Klein. God, for "He gave me hope when hope was gone, He gave me strength to journey on...." (*Les Miserables*)

We, Darla and Valerie, want to thank the following: Kathy Drehobl for her wonderful advice and encouragement. Marsha Dunn Klein, for taking us under her wing and providing us with invaluable information regarding the publishing process. Tami Hirasawa for her clinical knowledge and thorough reviews of the book. Kathy Rampy for her parental perspective and eye for grammar errors. Kristin Wallace, for her knack for organization and gift for helping us sound more like humans and less like OTs. Imaginart—especially Cindy, Nancy and Christine—for their help. And, the children and their families we have had the privilege to serve and who are the very reason for this book.

Valerie Pieraccini

and

Darla K. Vance

Contents

Caregiver Articles: Hand Skills in Daily Activities

Caregiver Articles: Adaptations for Hand Activities

Activities: 6 Months to 1½ Years

Activities: 1½ to 3 Years

Activities: 3 to 5 Years

Appendix

Glossary

References

About the Authors

Foreword

The trend in provision of early intervention services is to focus on family-centered programs in the natural environment. Pediatric therapists and educators have had to learn to work in partnership with parents to provide optimum programs for children. *Handprints: Home Programs for Hand Skills* authors, Valerie Pieraccini and Darla Vance, offer a wonderful support for parents, therapists and early interventionists who are providing services in the home as well as the classroom. They have done a beautiful job in celebrating and supporting parents in this clear, creative and informative book!

Handprints makes sense of the world of fine motor skills without the usual therapy jargon that can be so confusing to families. This book offers understandable explanations of hand development as a foundation for the creative activities offered. Fine motor components are analyzed from hand design to grasp, from release to manipulation, from strength to stability. Each component is described as it relates to typical development in parent-friendly terms, not in therapy-specific jargon.

Handprints is written in a child-friendly fashion. We know children have individual and unique learning styles. Some children learn by watching and imitating. Some learn by listening. Some learn by experiencing. Others learn by combining these styles. The hand activities provided in this book offer a multitude of different sensory experiences for the child. Activities are suggested in the context of everyday activities in which the child participates. Activities stimulate all different senses to support the learning styles of each child in creative and playful ways.

Parents and other caregivers also need their learning styles supported! When we, as early educators and pediatric therapists, realize that parents, too, have different learning styles, we expand our presentation of home therapy programs to include multi-sensory information. Parents tell us they appreciate these variations in presentation and learn more comfortably when their individual learning style is appreciated. *Handprints* provides clear and friendly explanations of the development of the hand and its function in a visually comfortable way. The authors realize many families appreciate a written handout to support the therapeutic explanation shared in the therapy setting or classroom. Many illustrations add to the visual clarity and support the visual learning styles of readers. The authors also challenge the readers to try some of these activities themselves in an effort to help them more sensitively understand the child's fine motor learning challenges.

We know parents are busy! Families are on the go more than ever before. They let us know that it is often difficult to find the time and energy to carry out therapy activities in the home. To add one or two or three new activities into the daily schedule can be overwhelming. *Handprints* gives parents short explanations of the "whys" of the activities as well as the information necessary to creatively incorporate the "therapeutic suggestions" into the family's normal routine. The "whys" give the parents the reasons for the activities. The "overwhelm" is decreased when the activities fit so nicely into the natural environment and daily routine of the family.

Gone are the days of lots of direct therapy. The funding just is not there. As funding becomes increasingly more difficult, we can no longer treat liberally and expect to be funded. We need to meet the child and family, evaluate the needs of the child within the context of the nurturing family, offer some direct treatment and then provide extensive home programs. Home programs are the way we can impact more children and their families. Funding sources have begun to require that pediatric therapies must take place in the home or the environment most natural for that child. *Handprints* provides therapists with a wealth of ideas for therapeutic explanations and child-centered or family-centered activities. These authors clearly understand that therapists can guide, but parents will make the biggest impact on the child.

Valerie Pieraccini and Darla Vance have certainly left their "handprints" on the field of pediatric occupational therapy. I wish them well.

Marsha Dunn Klein

Introduction

Through history, the handprint has been used as a symbol of both our uniqueness and our commonality. From cave walls to Hollywood sidewalks to preschool classrooms around the world, the handprint symbolizes humanity. The handprint also represents an essential component of our functionality. It is the physical representation of our ability to impact our environment by touching, grasping, pulling, pushing and manipulating it.

Handprints: Home Programs for Hand Skills is a manual that contains reproducible articles and activities which focus on the development of children's hand skills.

Populations for Whom This Book Was Designed

Handprints is a teaching tool designed especially for parents and caregivers of children with special needs whose chronological or developmental ages range from early infancy to five years. The material in *Handprints* addresses the needs of children with mild to moderate fine motor delays, such as children with Down syndrome, Spina Bifida, prematurity or global developmental delays. Some material is appropriate for use with more motorically involved populations such as children with neurological impairments like mild cerebral palsy or acquired head injury. Activities and many articles in *Handprints* can also be used with the child whose development is normal.

How Parents/Caregivers Are Provided This Information

This manual is intended to complement and enhance the early intervention and preschool program professional's instruction to the parent/caregiver. The child's occupational therapist (OT) or certified occupational therapist assistant (COTA) is best qualified to identify the child's needs in the area of hand skills and to match the information in *Handprints* with these needs. Along with the professional's verbal advice and physical demonstration, articles and activities from *Handprints* can be disseminated to mirror treatment priorities established in initial and ongoing assessments in therapy.

Educating the Parent and the Importance of Parent/Caregiver Involvement

Parent/caregiver participation is the most important factor in how much and how quickly the child progresses. As OTs working in a pediatric clinic where children are typically seen one hour per week, we are acutely aware of the importance of the parent's role in the child's development. With parent involvement, the child's progress is usually consistent and dependable, almost creating its own momentum. Without parent involvement, the child's progress is limited. The same skills are practiced again and again, and the child never seems to move forward. The child, parent and therapist can become easily frustrated. This difference in rate of skill acquisition occurs because the parent and child have more opportunities throughout the week to work on activities facilitating hand skill development. The typical one-hour-a-week therapy session can help establish motor patterns or set the stage for learning. It cannot, however, provide the practice and repetition the child needs to learn proficiency in a new skill. Yet, many families have limitations on their time, especially when children are part of a single-parent family or a family where both parents have jobs. Just taking the child to his therapy sessions is time consuming. Parents need information that can be easily and quickly read and that is highly relevant to their child's needs.

Handprints contains articles of four or fewer pages that explain why each hand skill is important for the child to learn. Each article emphasizes the importance of a particular hand skill as it relates to functional daily activities in a child's life. By matching the skill and function, the parent/caregiver can more fully understand the purpose and importance of the hand skill. This awareness will help parents make working on their child's hand skills a priority. As an adjunct to the hand skill articles, the activity pages provide simple activities using materials that can be readily found in most homes. Each activity demonstrates how to encourage development of a particular hand skill. Combined, the hand skill articles and activity pages provide a comprehensive picture for the parent—the *why* and *how* of hand skills.

It has been our experience that most parents are enthusiastic and appreciative when they are offered the chance to learn more about their developing child. Information on why hand skills are important and how they can best be practiced at home helps parents gain knowledge and become better observers of their children's abilities. As an added benefit, a parent who learns to better observe his child will probably be more confident in asking questions. Participation encourages parents to feel good about their role in their child's progress. They do not need to passively wait for change to occur in therapy: their love and dedication to work to improve their child's skills is the catalyst for change. This emphasis on parent and caregiver education is consistent with the current trend of working with the child in his natural environment. Children benefit greatly from parents or caregivers who are empowered to practice needed skills in the setting where the child is most comfortable.

Rationale for Included Topics

It was not until we were involved in the literature review for this book that we discovered the many different definitions of the term *fine motor skill*. Some sources categorize fine motor skills as vision and all upper extremity movement and function, while others focus only on intrinsic muscle use in the hands. Although this disparity is frustrating, it does bring up the point that nothing—not even one of the cornerstone concepts in occupational therapy—is without its gray areas. Myers (1992) implies that activities involving the use of the hands and fingers that are called fine motor are not necessarily fine motor activities because they do not involve movements of the intrinsic muscles of the metacarpophalangeal joints. Reed and Sanderson (1983) broadly define fine motor skills as the ability or performance in which discrete, specialized muscle groups or systems are used. In a resource book for normal development, Alexander, Boehme and Cupps (1993) include upper extremity, hand and visual development under the heading of fine motor development. Another source frequently used by OTs, *The Peabody Developmental Motor Scales: Fine Motor Subtest* (Folio, Fewell, 1983), includes skills such as grasping, hand use, eye-hand coordination and manual dexterity. The specific test items include activities that involve reaching and bilateral coordination as well as tool use. Charlotte Exner, an expert in fine motor performance and function, describes fine motor skills as being synonymous with hand skills (Case-Smith, et al., 1996). Exner defines hand skills as movement "patterns including basic reach, grasp, carry, release and the more complex skills of in-hand manipulation and bilateral hand use"(1996, p. 268).

Keeping all of this in mind, our goal in creating *Handprints* was to develop a comprehensive resource book on the topics surrounding hand skills. These topics had to include the subjects that OTs focus on when discussing a child's hand skills with his parents. Since the definition of a fine motor skill/hand skill is somewhat conflicting, we felt freed from having to adhere to any one definition. By choosing a broader perspective of the term, we have been able to provide more information for therapists to disseminate to their clients' families. You'll find that this book includes many articles that address a number of skills and adaptations that impact hand skills, but are not typically viewed as fine motor skills. The "Hand Skills and Related Topics" and the "Adaptations for Hand Activities" sections include articles that address shoulder strength and stability, trunk stability, presentation of a task and positioning the child. We have included articles that are more anatomic and preparatory in nature. For example, the "Hand Skills and Related Topics" section includes articles on hand structure and upper extremity weightbearing. We also included sensory-type observations because they relate closely to the child's ability to use his hands in a functional way. Motor planning, haptic sense, environmental adaptations and providing the "just right" challenge are examples of article topics in the "Hand Skills and Related Topics" and "Adaptations for Hand Activities" sections.

Throughout history, OTs have been concerned with what is functional and meaningful to their clients. They have highlighted the importance of gaining independence in one's activities of daily living, as well as one's work and leisure (Punwar, 1988). For this reason, we included articles to educate the parent/caregiver on how hand skills relate to a child's daily activities. "Hand Skills in Daily Activities" includes topics that range from drinking to signing.

Activity analysis is also a fundamental part of occupational therapy. Fully understanding the activity—and all of its components—is the first consideration when working with a client (Hopkins, Smith, 1988). In the "Adaptations for Hand Activities" section, we have attempted to guide the parent in making simple observations about his child's performance in an activity so that the parent can make appropriate changes. The "Adaptations for Hand Activities" section also provides us with a venue to pass on helpful lessons we have learned from gifted teachers in our lives, namely the children and families with whom we have worked. These articles include information from a variety of facets of life, not necessarily those ordinarily considered to be under the umbrella of hand skills, but affecting them just the same.

The topic of cognition is not included in *Handprints*. We recognize the role cognitive ability plays in hand skills, particularly when impairment is present, and especially when the child has profound mental retardation. Parents may provide stimulation to ensure that their child develops to the best of his ability; however, prognosis for the acquisition of complex hand skills for a child with severe cognitive impairment may remain poor. Children with mild cognitive impairment may also experience delays in their skills. How a child's cognitive skills affect his hand skills should be discussed in a one-on-one and compassionate manner with the parent/caregiver.

Similarly, vision—in terms of visual acuity—is not highlighted here. Visual impairment can have an adverse effect on hand skills. Infants who are blind from birth, but have no other physical disabilities, are known to have delayed self-initiated movements. In this manual, however, vision is discussed in terms of its functional role in hand skills, such as described in the "Hand Skills and Related Topics" articles on eye-hand coordination and visual perception.

Handprints attempts to provide a comprehensive, but not cumbersome, tool that deals with the discrepancies in literature without being misleading or confusing. Rather, it is meant to empower the clinician and the clients' families and caregivers by providing information that can be easily used without compromising accuracy.

How to Use This Book

The text in *Handprints* is divided into two main categories: *Caregiver Articles* and *Activities.* The *Caregiver Articles* contain the sections "Hand Skills and Related Topics," "Hand Skills in Daily Activities" and "Adaptations for Hand Activities." Each article in the "Hand Skills and Related Topics" section provides a definition and description of a particular hand skill, an explanation of the development of that skill and an example of how that skill affects daily function. Each of the articles in the "Hand Skills in Daily Activities" section thoroughly describes the major components of one activity of daily living and how that activity progresses as the child's hand skills develop. The "Adaptations for Hand Activities" section provides general guidelines and suggestions on how to change an activity, environment or attitude to allow the child to be more successful. Each of the *Caregiver Articles* has a clinical title in the upper corner to help the therapist quickly ascertain clinical content of the article.

The *Activities* section contains specific activities arranged according to developmental age. Each activity lists the materials that are needed, explains how to do the activity, describes how to make the activity easier or harder and briefly defines the hand skills that are addressed.

The *Appendix* contains two charts and a checklist to be used by the therapist in conjunction with the articles and activities. Also included is a toy list which may be given to parents at the therapist's discretion. The "Which Activity, Which Hand Skills?" chart and the "Which Activity, Which Hand Skills in Daily Activities?" chart help the therapist clearly delineate which activities should be given with which hand skill article. The checklist provides space to record which handouts have been given to the family of each child. The list "Toys, Toys and More Toys" provides information on toys that can be purchased and the hand skills they promote. The *Glossary* provides definitions of hand skills referred to in the *Handprints* text.

Clearly drawn illustrations throughout *Handprints* provide clarification of a specific hand position, tool or activity suggested in the text. All articles and activities in this book include an age range at the upper corner of the page. This number reflects a child's developmental or skill level age rather than a child's chronological age. The age range provided is not necessarily when that skill begins to emerge, but when it is appropriate in the child's development to give this information to the parent. For example, play begins in early infancy when only basic hand skills are available to the child. However, the article, "Come Out and Play With Me," (page 78) which looks at hand skills in play, is more appropriate for the 1-year-old child and older because it is at this time that the child's play becomes more diverse due to increased motor competency. It should be emphasized that these age ranges are just general guidelines. Decisions regarding how and when to give out this information should never be based solely on these age ranges. The most effective approach to utilizing *Handprints* should incorporate the therapist's experiences and knowledge of the specific needs and interests of the child regardless of that child's developmental age.

It is also important to consider the dynamics of the specific family involved when determining how best to present this information. If appropriate, the clinical title of the exercise and the developmental age range can be removed from the top of the page for the parent's copy by simply adjusting the paper on the copier or covering that space with other paper when copying. Also, keep in mind that each parent's learning style and learning curve is different. Therefore, it might be appropriate to give a home program packet that includes both parent articles and activities to one family, while another family might do better with an article one week and an activity the next.

The following paragraphs provide further explanation and detail about each section's contents and purpose.

Caregiver Articles: Hand Skills and Related Topics

This section (page 9) provides 19 parent/caregiver articles on various hand skills and skills that directly affect hand skills. It explains in simple terms what a specific skill is, how it develops, and how it relates to function. When defining the hand skill, clinical terms have been avoided as much as possible. Often, examples have been used that the parent can relate to or observe. For example, in "Head and Shoulders, Trunk and Hands" (page 32), the parent is asked to remember or imagine what it is like to write while in a moving car. Although some developmental ages are provided in the text, the emphasis is on the sequence of events that occur in development and how each step depends on the other. The articles often provide examples of how the particular skill becomes increasingly important as the child grows older. For example, "As the Hand Turns" (page 43) explains that in-hand manipulation is needed to tie shoestrings and buckle a belt—skills that do not appear until the child is much older. This emphasis helps families understand the importance of addressing these primary skills early in their child's life and not waiting until there is a problem in school or with self-help skills later.

Caregiver Articles: Hand Skills in Daily Activities

This section (page 63) provides 10 parent/caregiver articles that address the relationship between hand skills and activities of a child's daily living. Each article explains one specific daily living activity, the hand skills involved and what each developmental stage of the activity looks like. Although few people need a definition of a daily living skill (such as eating, drinking or cutting with scissors), examples have been given to help families relate to their child's attempts to learn the task. Again, when defining the hand skills necessary for the task, clinical terms have been avoided as much as possible. As in the previous section, some developmental ages are provided in the text, but the emphasis is on the sequence of skill development necessary to perform the task.

Caregiver Articles: Adaptations for Hand Activities

This section (page 97) provides 11 parent/caregiver articles that suggest generalized adaptations which are not specific to any one activity and may be used with activities that are not in *Handprints*. These articles recommend how to change the tools, setup or environment for a child to be successful, yet challenged, during almost any task. Children with typical or atypical development can benefit from some of these suggestions. For example, "Writing on the Wall" (page 124) explains that some activities can be enhanced by being moved from a horizontal surface to a vertical surface. Playing on a vertical surface is important for all children to develop needed musculature for writing. Some articles are more limited to a certain population's needs. "If You Are a Lefty and You Know It, Clap Your Hands" (page 126) suggests how to adapt activities using tools for the child who prefers left-handedness.

Activities

This section (page 131), broken up by age level, contains 30 fun ways for parents to play with their children while addressing the development of hand skills. To make it easier and more practical for parents, all materials for the activities are easily obtained if not already present in the home. Some activities have an end product, such as a plant in "Green Thumb," (page 162), while others can be done just for the sheer fun of it.

The "Materials" section lists the materials needed to complete the activity. This allows the parent to plan ahead, gathering all materials needed prior to the child's involvement.

The "How to" section describes, in order, each step in the activity. Some of the directions are preceded by a "Preparation" statement, which informs the parent of any work that needs to be completed before the child can participate.

The "Adaptations" section offers ideas for parents to make this activity easier if the child is struggling with the task. It also offers suggestions to make the activity harder if the child is not being sufficiently challenged.

The "Why" section helps the parent recognize the priority skills which are addressed in the activity. Each skill is defined simply, followed by examples of functional tasks that incorporate the skill. To make this section less overwhelming, only the top four hand skills for each activity are identified, even though the activity might involve other noteworthy skills.

Finally, the "Comments" section is the therapist's chance to further adapt or customize this activity for the specific child for whom the activity was chosen.

Activities are organized into three different age ranges: 6 months to 1½ years, 1½ to 3 years and 3 to 5 years. It should be noted that because a list of adaptations which make the activities easier or harder has been included with each activity, some activities placed in higher age categories could be simplified to make them more appropriate for younger age levels, and vice versa. For example, although the activity "Feely Box" is placed in the age category of 6 months to 1½ years, by simply using the adaptation to identify familiar toys hidden in the prepared box, this activity could be used with older children in the developmental age range of 3 to 5 years.

Combining the Caregiver Articles With Activities

This manual should read like a recipe book. The professional is the chef who plans what recipes to use to create a meal experience. The chef's knowledge, experience and intuition allow her to know what side dishes go with what main course, as well as what beverage best complements the meal. In much the same way, the OT or COTA, with her educational background, clinical experience and gut instinct, knows a child's specific areas of need and is able to choose a hand skill article that best reflects that area of need. Furthermore, the therapist is able to complement that skill by providing an activity that reinforces the skill. For example, if the child has poor shoulder strength, the therapist might first provide the parent with a copy of "The Shoulder Bone Is Connected to the Wrist Bone," an article discussing the importance and development of shoulder strength and stability. After referring to the "Which Activity, Which Hand Skills?" chart in the Appendix, the therapist could choose to complete the home program packet by including copies of "Golf Ball Roll" and "Paint Your World with Water," activities that incorporate upper extremity and shoulder strengthening.

In another example, a child may be struggling with dressing. The OT can provide the parent with the article "1, 2, Buckle My Shoe," which looks at the hand skills involved in dressing. Taking it a step further, the therapist, who recognizes that the child's problems are due to his difficulties with bilateral coordination and precision grasping, can then provide the articles "Hand in Hand" and "At Your Fingertips," which address bilateral coordination and the precision grasp, respectively. Finally, after referring to the "Which Activity, Which Hand Skill?" chart, the home program packet can be completed by sharing the activity "Putting money in the bank" with the parent, which highlights both of these needed skills affecting the child's ability to dress independently.

Appendix

The appendix includes the following sections:

Charts

Two charts are provided as a guide to show which articles are compatible with which activities. One chart shows how the first section of the Caregiver Articles, "Hand Skills and Related Topics" relates to the activities, while the other chart shows which activities incorporate different aspects of the second section of the Caregiver Articles, "Hand Skills in Daily Activities."

Checklist

Along with the charts, a checklist is provided to help keep track of articles and activities and the exact dates they were given to the parent.

Toy List

The handout "Toys, Toys and More Toys" is designed to help the parent purchase toys that address specific hand skills. It organizes popular toys into five different developmental age categories and lists the two primary hand skills each toy promotes. Each age category represents when the toy will first provide a challenge for the child, yet still allow for success. Many of the toys are appropriate past the age for which they are first mentioned.

Glossary

The glossary provides definitions of hand skills in parent-friendly terms. Each definition includes examples of how these skills are used in the child's daily life. These definitions are consistent with those listed in the "Why" section at the end of each activity.

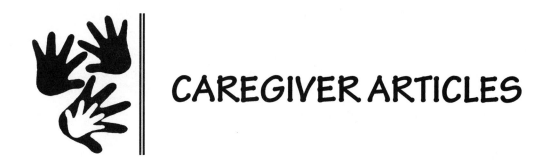

CAREGIVER ARTICLES

HAND SKILLS AND RELATED TOPICS

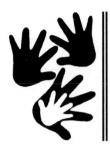

A HAND-SOME DESIGN

As a parent, you probably never thought there was any reason for you to know the names of all the bones in the hand, all the muscles that move the bones and all the nerves that supply the muscles. That is, unless you were playing a game of knowledge such as Trivial Pursuit® with your children. It *is* important, however, for you as a parent to understand how all these parts of the hand work together for grasp, release, manipulation and other skilled movements so that you can be a better observer of your child's hand skills. You just might not need to remember all the names!

The structure of the hand allows for a variety of movement.

The hand has a truly amazing design. By being mobile and pliable, it can produce many combinations of movement. By blending movement from the wrist, palm and fingers, the hand can mold itself to the shape of an infinite number of objects. It can squeeze an exercise handgrip with a force up to 100 pounds. It can also remove a thread from a garment. No other body part is so adaptable.

To learn about the hand, let's start at the wrist and proceed to the fingertips. Like the shoulder and elbow, the wrist has an effect on hand function by placing the hand in the right place at the right time. The position of the wrist also affects how well the muscles of the hand work. If you bend your wrist forward or backward as far as you can, you will notice that trying to make your thumb, index finger and middle finger move, as if writing with a pen, is very difficult. That's because the muscles that make these small movements for writing work best when the wrist is slightly bent upward with the pinky side of the hand resting on the table. This position sets up the thumb and fingers to work well together, like when you sign your name. The wrist is also where the group of muscles that is responsible for large movements of the hand passes through from the forearm. These muscles are responsible for movements like rocking your hand from side to side when you wave.

Now look at the palm. Despite the thickness of the skin, it has many creases that allow you to make a fist and do other movements. Other features on the surface of the palm are two pads on each side, one under the pinky and one under the thumb. Under these pads are the muscles responsible for the small movements of the hand. If you put your pinky and thumb together, like when gesturing the number three, you can see these muscles as they become more pronounced with the wrinkling of the hand. Now with your palm facing toward you, open and close your hands and then cup your hands. See how much movement your palm allows? The palm can be completely flat to pat cookie dough or it can create a concave surface like when you cup your hand to gather crumbs from a table. This flexibility is due to the design of the bones in the hand, which make up three sets of arches. These arches give the fingers a large range of movement so they can grasp many sizes of objects. This allows the hand to grasp that loose thread or squeeze the exercise hand grip with a strong grasp.

Now look at the fingers. Because they are always involved in grasping objects, it is the fingers of our children that always seem to be getting pinched or caught. The fingers' main purpose is to grasp, hold or release objects. Each finger has its own important role, yet all the fingers work together.

The thumb is very different from the others. The fact that it has only two joints and is quite a bit shorter is just the beginning. The thumb has many more movements than the other fingers. Although it can move more independently, its main function is to work with the other fingers by providing an opposing force to hold objects. It would be very difficult for your child to button a shirt or tie a shoelace without his thumb.

The index finger also is very mobile and can work somewhat independently. See how easily our young children isolate the index finger to poke into every hole available? Like the thumb, it is almost always involved when the hand is grasping an object.

The middle finger sometimes replaces the index finger during pinch grasps, like when you pick up a raisin. The longer the finger, the stronger that finger is, which makes the middle finger the strongest. Therefore, the middle finger is often involved in picking up objects and manipulating them.

The ring and pinky fingers are the weakest, but they're included in power grips, like when you need to open a jar of jelly for your child's peanut butter sandwich.

So the design of the hand is truly amazing. It allows us to adapt our hands to fit all types of objects. No wonder we use them to do so much.

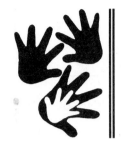

YOU'VE GOT THE WHOLE WORLD IN YOUR HAND

If you have ever heard the term "fine motor," you might have thought that the speaker was referring to an expensive automobile! The term fine motor can be confusing because it is not something you think or talk about in your typical day. In the context of the human body, fine motor refers to the movements of the small muscles of the body.

Which body parts do you imagine have large muscles and which parts have small muscles? You have large muscles in your trunk, legs and arms. These large muscles are called on to perform large and powerful movements of your body, such as running, doing a cartwheel and lifting weights. In contrast, the small muscles of your body, like the muscles in your hands, are called upon to do the more skilled and precise movements, such as drawing a picture, cutting out a valentine, unbuttoning a button or turning a nut on a bolt. Both sets of muscles are important to

Buttoning requires small muscle movements from both hands.

the development of hand skills. The large muscles keep the body stable, while the small muscles actually perform the specialized movements needed to accomplish a detailed task. Did you realize that when you reach for a cup in your cupboard, the first muscles to activate are

14

actually in your legs? Your body is creating a steady base to counter-act your arm moving away from your body. With the stability provided by the large muscles in your legs and trunk, you are able to use the small muscles in your hand to grasp the handle on your china cup.

In the hand, you have two different sizes of muscles. First, you have large muscles coming from your upper arm into your hand—often referred to as the "extrinsic" muscles. These are the muscles responsible for movements like kneading bread dough, carrying a suitcase or waving to a friend. Second, you have the small muscles that start just below your wrist—often referred to as the "intrinsic" muscles. These are the muscles responsible for movements like sealing a plastic bag, lifting a pin from a pincushion or picking up a french fry. The intrinsic muscles are key to the development of fine motor skills because their main purpose is skill and precision—both important aspects of using your hands.

Fine motor skills are often considered to be the same as hand skills because most of this detailed work requiring small muscles happens in the hands. With respect to hand skills, there are a number of things to observe in your child's play that will tell you how she is using her hands. How does your child reach for an object or toy? How does she grasp the toy? Does she use all her fingers together or can some fingers move by themselves? How does your child let go of the object? How does she turn or move a toy in her hands to examine it? How does she use both hands together to interact with a toy? How does she use a tool, such as working with a shovel in the sand?

What can you do to help your child learn these important hand skills? There are certain basic skills that, once learned, will encourage overall better hand skills in your child. Let's look at these basic skills: they all can be seen when you write.

When writing, notice how your wrist stays in a straight position. Now try writing with your wrist bent forward or flexed. It is very difficult and uncomfortable to make smooth and controlled movements in this flexed position. A straight wrist allows a balance between the small movements of straightening and bending the fingers. This can also be seen when you roll a ball of play dough with your fingertips or when you type on a keyboard. Your child needs to learn how to keep a straightened, or extended, wrist during play.

When writing, also notice how your palm curves toward the pencil and how your index finger, middle finger and thumb form a circular shape. This arching or cupping enables your hand to curve around objects like a pencil. It also allows your hand to bring the thumb to the other fingers on the same hand, as seen when you pick up a small object like a pushpin. Your child needs to learn how to arch or cup her hand instead of having a flat hand.

Arching enables the hand to curve around the pencil.

Finally, when writing, notice how your index finger, middle finger and thumb actually control the movement of the pencil, as your ring and pinky fingers appear to be resting in your palm. Your thumb, middle and index fingers are more skillful while the ring and pinky fingers are tucked in the palm to provide stability. You can also clearly see this separation of the different sides of the hand in activities such as fastening your watch or putting a barrette in your hair. Your child needs to learn to use the skilled side of the hand.

So as your child develops and gains strength and control of both the large and small muscles of the body, you will see a big improvement in how she can use her hands. Encouraging your child to learn a few basic skills will help her develop better control of the small muscles. This will open a whole new world of possibilities of what she can do with her hands. And someday your child may be replacing the spark plugs in the "fine motor" of that expensive automobile.

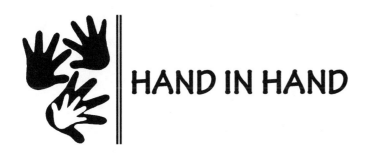

HAND IN HAND

The list is endless. You steer a car. You swing a golf club. You type a letter. You pick up a baby from a crib. You put on a sweater. You staple papers together. You clap for a performance. You flatten cookie dough with a rolling pin. You put a ponytail in a little girl's hair. These are just a few of the many tasks where you use bilateral coordination of your hands.

Bilateral coordination is the ability to use the two sides of your body together in a coordinated manner. Bilateral coordination of the eyes allows you to read a book, and bilateral coordination of the legs allows you to walk. Bilateral coordination is possible because of a process in the brain, called bilateral integration, that coordinates sensations from both sides of your body. The combination of these sensations, especially from the skin, joints, muscles and eyes, provides an internal image of the body and how the parts relate to each other. In a young child, this information eventually leads to an understanding of how to use body parts, such as her hands, together well when she plays with toys.

Since bilateral coordination of the arms develops before the legs, you may first notice your child using the opposite sides of her body together when she starts bringing a toy or bottle to her mouth. However, a child must develop many skills to go from being able to hold a bottle in both hands to being able to do the list of tasks from the beginning of this article. To use her hands together well requires that your child plan her movements, including coordinating each hand's timing of movement in space. It also requires her to remember the sequence of movements necessary for the task. If you ever watch someone knitting, the movement of the knitter's hands appears to have a rhythm.

HAND IN HAND (continued)

There are several ways you use your hands together, but they generally fall into three categories. A child typically is able to use her hands in all three of these ways by her third birthday. One way you use your hands together is when you hold an object with both hands acting in unison. The approach is called unison. Your hands often mirror each other's movement or position. This is the first way an infant uses her hands together when she reaches for or holds a toy, because an infant's movements are very symmetrical. You use this approach, too, when you carry a large object such as a beach ball or box.

Another way you use your hands together is when one hand holds or stabilizes the object while the other hand carries out the activity of exploring or manipulating it. This approach is called differentiated. You may notice that your child can hold a toy with one hand while poking at it with another hand. If so, your child is now able to use the two sides of her body differently. When you write a letter, you use this approach. You use one hand to write while stabilizing the paper with the other.

Using one hand to hold the paper and one to color requires differentiated bilateral coordination.

A third way to use your hands together is to use both hands to do different but complementary movements at the same time. It is no surprise that this approach is called complementary. When your child buttons her shirt, one hand pushes the button through the hole while the other hand pulls the cloth over the button. When you type on the computer, your fingers hit different keys while working together to produce words in a document.

18

HAND IN HAND (continued)

So you see, the ability to use your two hands together well is not just child's play. It is important for the most basic activities of your daily routine throughout your whole life. And the list of how you use your hands together is truly endless. You toss a salad. You shake out a rug. You hit a ball with a baseball bat. You rake the yard. You put a lid on a pickle jar. . . .

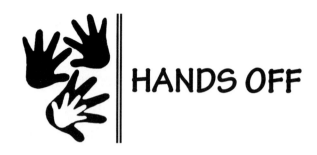

HANDS OFF

If you have ever seen a professional juggler, you can truly appreciate the art and fluidity of the movement of his hands. With his arms in constant motion, the performer is able to grasp and release the ball or apple so quickly that it's hard to separate one movement from the other. This is a perfect example of the effortless and flowing movement of well-coordinated eye and hand skills.

Your hands are tools that allow you to interact with your world. Most of the time, your hands are involved in grasping—or bringing your fingers toward your palms—to secure an object like a hairbrush or apple. This flexing or bending movement of your fingers is stronger and more frequently used than the act of straightening your fingers. In an infant, grasp actually develops before release. Release—or letting go of an object—first occurs reflexively in the young infant. When a child is as young as 3 weeks of age, with a slight touch to the back of his hand, he will open it, spread his fingers and drop a clutched toy. Through these early reflexes, the child is able to gradually learn the movements required to release an object. Eventually, the child learns to use purposeful releases to replace the more primitive reflexive releases.

At around 6 months of age, as the child mouths and handles toys with both hands, you can observe the beginnings of this more mature release.

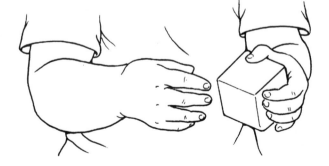

Moving the block from one hand to the other requires release as well as grasp.

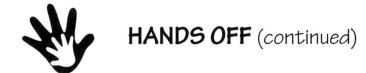

He might hold the toy in his mouth, letting one hand drop away. The child might also release an object from one hand by pulling it out with the other. He will also be able to release an object by using the surface of a table to help roll the object out of his hands. Around the same time, as the child plays on his tummy with his hands open, he is learning how to extend or straighten his fingers.

Since the child is still learning how to straighten his fingers in a controlled way, he will start by throwing or flinging an object from his hand. Parents usually have no difficulty recognizing this stage. Mealtimes most often require a tarp on the floor and a major cleanup! Next, the child will be able to have a controlled release by supporting his hand on a table surface when he releases a piece of food onto his tray. Eventually, at around 1½ to 2 years of age, the child will gain more control in straightening his fingers. He will no longer need a table surface when he releases a block or peg. He is now able to stack blocks, then remove his fingers with just enough pressure that the tower doesn't fall. He is also beginning to be able to place simple shapes into a shape sorter or release a raisin into a small opening in a container with precision and grace.

So when your child announces that he would like to be a knife or flame thrower when he grows up, be thankful that you've had a hand in teaching him how to grasp and release with accuracy!

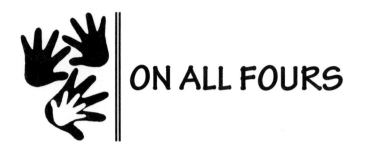

ON ALL FOURS

Have you ever done a push-up or been in a yoga position where you put weight on your hands and arms? Although it might not have felt good at the time, the benefits gained from bearing weight on your arms are many. In this position you are building muscle strength and increasing bone density in your back and arms. This is also true for the developing child. Weightbearing on the arms and hands helps prepare the young child for large muscle movements and for the development of hand skills.

At 4 months of age, a child is usually able to prop himself up on his elbows when he lies on his stomach to look at a toy. Around 6 months, the child begins to push up even higher by straightening his arms. Eventually, he can assume a position on hands and knees. Prior to crawling, the child will practice shifting his weight over his arms by reaching for toys and rocking back and forth. He may begin crawling on his hands and knees prior to 9 months. During this time of development, most parents are unaware that these activities are also preparing the child's hands for more difficult tasks such as writing and cutting with scissors.

When a child puts weight on his forearms or hands, he is strengthening and, consequently, stabilizing his shoulders. Stability at the shoulder is very important for the arm—specifically the hand—to have a steady base on which to work. When he bears weight on straightened arms, the child begins to stretch muscles of the arm that previously have not been used. He also begins to strengthen and gain control of his arm muscles when he bends and straightens his arms to raise and lower himself. These strengthened muscles in the shoulders, arms,

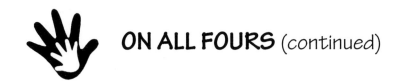

wrists and hands will later be used when he writes on a chalkboard or paints on an easel.

As the child reaches for toys while on his hands and knees, one arm must take all the weight while the other reaches. This experience encourages coordination between the arms to work separately but still together as a team. This coordination between the arms will be essential for more complex tasks such as cutting paper with scissors or twisting the cap off of a jar.

When a child moves from being on his hands and knees to sitting, he curves or cups the palms of his hands to maintain his balance. This balance reaction begins to strengthen the muscles of the palms used to curve around an object like a baseball, or to cup the palm in order to manipulate a piece of chalk.

When he crawls with a toy in his hand, the child usually holds the object with the thumb, index finger and middle finger while he puts his weight on the pinky side of his hand. This simple act teaches the child to use the two sides of the hands separately. Eventually, he will use the thumb, index and middle fingers to push, poke, turn or grasp objects while he curls the pinky side of his hand into his palm.

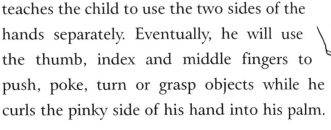

Even though walking is an exciting milestone, you may want to resist the temptation to encourage your child to walk too early.

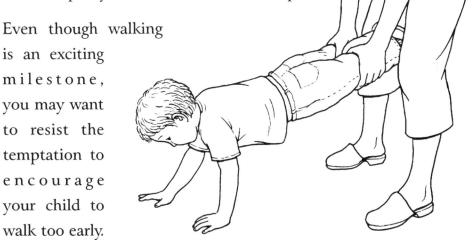

Weightbearing on arms during wheelbarrow walking.

ON ALL FOURS (continued)

Remember that your child will benefit from more time spent bearing weight on his arms. Even after your child has started walking, provide him with opportunities to get back on the ground and put weight on his arms. This will help him develop better hand skills to explore and manipulate the world around him. So as you encourage walking, remember to encourage "wheelbarrow" walking too!

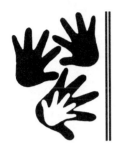

THE SHOULDER BONE IS CONNECTED TO THE WRIST BONE

Imagine a large construction crane at work. If the crane is not stabilized on the ground, the extended arm will not have a sturdy base to work from. Consequently, the crane will have poor control and precision. The same situation is true of the human arm. You need to have a stable trunk as well as the ability to stabilize your shoulders in order to use your hands efficiently.

Early in development, a baby develops shoulder and trunk strength when he is placed on his tummy and pushes his arms into the surface to lift up his head. Around 4 months of age, the child is able to prop himself on his elbows when lying on his tummy to look at a toy. Shortly, the child is able to push himself up even higher by

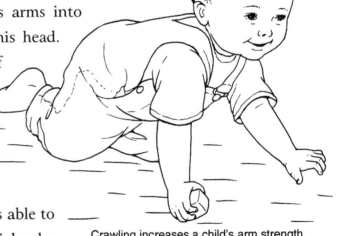

Crawling increases a child's arm strength.

straightening his arms while lying on his tummy and then shifting his weight from one side to the other to free up one arm for reaching. Soon after, the baby will push himself up into a hands-and-knees stance, eventually rocking and playing in this position. Around the 7- to 9-month period, the baby will push up into a sitting position, using his arms, and crawl on his hands and knees. Eventually, the baby will pull himself up into a standing position using mainly his arms on a stable, raised object, such as a sofa or table.

SHOULDER CONNECTED TO THE WRIST BONE
(continued)

As you can see, the arms continue to gain more and more strength and control in each stage of development. Strength and control are necessary for large movements to be smooth, like when the older child draws on the chalkboard or spins a jump rope. Similarly, strength and control are needed in small movements, such as buttoning, writing and cutting. Children who miss certain stages of development, such as crawling, will sometimes have poor shoulder stability later in

Maintaining the arm away from the body when stacking blocks demonstrates good shoulder strength.

life—especially when tasks become more difficult. We are able to assess a child's shoulder stability by observing how he holds his arms in space and in relation to his body. Often, a child with poor shoulder stability will keep his arms close to his body in an effort to use his trunk for stability rather than being able to maintain a steady arm position away from his body. Watching a simple activity, such as a child stacking blocks, can tell you many things. Look at how high and with how much control the child is able to stack the blocks. Does his arm stay steady and can he control it well, or does his arm sway or move too quickly?

Your body is so amazingly connected that limitations in one area directly influence the efficiency of another area. Remember the lesson from the construction crane. No digging can happen without first creating a stable position on the ground for the base of the arm. Without stability in your shoulders, you cannot expect to have the kind of control you need at your fingertips to perform daily tasks and activities. Helping your child to develop stronger shoulder and arm muscles will allow him to use his arms and hands in many ways. Who knows, maybe someday he will even manage the controls of a large construction vehicle.

26

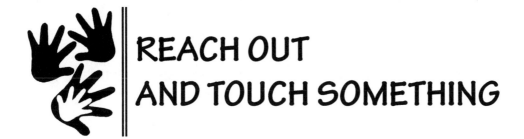

REACH OUT AND TOUCH SOMETHING

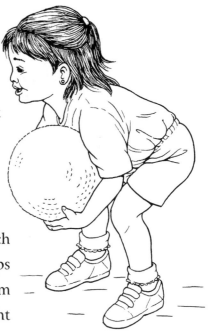

Reaching is an important skill in catching a ball.

A primary purpose of the hand is to shape itself around an object. This includes being able to grasp and release the object. The purpose of the arm is to take the hand to the object, at exactly the right time and place. Think about baseball. It takes tremendous cooperation between the arm and the hand to catch a baseball. The arm must get the hand in the right location to catch the ball, no matter how far a player jumps or runs to intercept the ball. The arm must have the hand there at just the right time. Because of the speed of the base-ball, seconds can make a difference in whether or not the player catches the ball. On top of all that, the hand also must be prepared to catch the baseball. Inside the mitt, the play-er's fingers will begin to close around the ball to catch it moments before actual contact.

Many things happen "behind the scenes" of the arm and hand that allow this awesome feat of reaching to take place. When you decide that you want to touch or hold an object with your hands, you must gather certain information. Typically, your vision locates the object. It also gives information about the object's size, shape and texture. By seeing what is in the environment around the object, it also helps you to anticipate what might happen when you reach for it. Vision allows you to plan the path your arm should follow to grasp the object with

27

your hand. It also allows you to shape your hand in preparation for grasping the object. Before reaching, you must also be aware of where your body is in space—particularly where your arm and hand are. This information, provided primarily through receptors in the muscles, joints and skin, tells you the position of your body in relation to your environment. As you reach, these receptors tell you where your arm is, as well as the speed and direction of your arm movements. So, just as the ball player is able to judge where the batter hit the ball in relation to where he is in the field, your child needs to know where he is in relationship to the toy he wants to get.

With the information you receive, your body is able to respond appropriately. You make adjustments in your posture in anticipation of reaching. This allows you to shift your weight without losing your balance. If the baseball player loses his balance and falls, he will not catch the ball. Likewise, your child must be able to maintain her balance to support the movement of her arms in reaching.

This information also allows you to plan and implement movements that are concise, so you don't waste energy. When you reach for the simple sake of reaching, there are multiple combinations of movement patterns that could be used. However, if there is a goal to win a baseball game, then the skilled athlete will use the most efficient movement pattern to catch the ball. His reach is very smooth and coordinated as his arm moves. In like manner, your child learns to use the most successful and efficient patterns of reach to get a toy. And, because no two situations are the same, your child will always need to adapt her movements according to the circumstances.

Amazingly, a young child has typically acquired much of these basic reaching skills by the age of 1½ years. After that age, these basic skills are refined through practice. With lots of practice, your child may even have the catch of a professional baseball player.

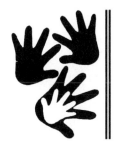

AT YOUR FINGERTIPS

Perhaps you remember plucking flower petals while saying, "Loves me, loves me not." Or maybe as a child you plucked the legs off of a grasshopper to see what would happen. Either way, you now remember what it looks like to use a precision grasp.

As you pick a small object off a table, observe your hand. As you reach toward the object, you create a space between your fingers and thumb. Notice that with different objects, your fingers and the space between your fingers look different. This shape between your fingers will change from a circular space when you use your fingertips to pick up a needle to more of an oval shape when you use your finger pads to pick up a penny. Because the needle is smaller than the penny, the fingers' and thumb's actions have to be more precise, requiring just the tips of the fingers. With the penny, which has a larger surface, the finger pads have better control. Also, when you need a firm grasp on a slightly larger object, you might use the thumb, index and middle finger to complete the activity, such as when you open a small twist-top container. Having a number of different types of precision grasps allows us to choose the most appropriate grasp for whatever we are doing.

These precision grasps develop over time as the child uses his hands in movement and in play. The newborn child has a reflex that causes his fingers to trap objects against the palm whenever an object is placed there. In the first few months, the infant will learn to

Creating a circular space between the index finger and thumb during a precision grasp.

grasp purposefully at toys using movement of his fingers toward the palm, but without involving the thumb. Eventually, the child will learn to include the thumb as he grasps with his whole hand, such as when he holds a teething biscuit. Around the child's sixth month, the beginning of precision grasp emerges. You may see him use his thumb, index finger and middle finger to hold a circular ring. As the child slowly gains refined control toward the ends of his fingers, you might see the 10-month-old pinch with the tip of his index finger and thumb. This allows him to pick up a piece of dry cereal with accuracy.

What characteristics make your fingers and thumb perfect for their role in a precision grasp? First of all, the fingertips and pads are very sensitive to touch sensations. This provides a great deal of information about the object. Another important characteristic is the structure of your hands. Because of how your fingers and thumb are positioned with their pads facing each other, they are able to move toward and with each other more easily. Also, the fingers and thumb can make small, controlled movements that allow you to easily turn or move a small item once it is in the hand. Can you imagine threading a needle using your toes? The foot is definitely not designed for such precision grasping!

Although you would think that you would have to use your eyes for a precision grasp, this is not necessarily the case. The most important thing in being able to use a precision grasp is knowing where the object is. The method of feeling for the object with your whole hand and then corralling it up to the index finger and thumb can work just as well as locating the object with your eyes. Either way, you can successfully use your index finger and thumb to pinch with precision to pick up a small object like a bead.

As your child matures and grows, these precision grasps will be increasingly important and necessary in more complex tasks, such as buttoning a vest, opening a toothpaste tube or using a pencil to draw a picture. With the future in mind, you can look at the bright side of learning a precision grasp as you watch your child picking apart your flowers or redesigning some poor insect!

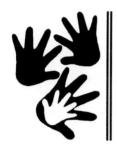

HEAD AND SHOULDERS, TRUNK AND HANDS

Have you ever tried to write when your feet were not supported, such as when you were sitting on a barstool? Without a place to stabilize your feet, and therefore your body, you tend to stabilize in other places. Some people attempt to stabilize themselves by tightly wrapping their feet around the stool legs. Others plant their forearms or wrists on the table, making it difficult to freely move their hand to write. Can you recall trying to write while you were in a moving car? With continual turns, stops and starts, it's difficult for your hand to remain steady on the paper. These examples illustrate just a few ways having an unstable trunk can affect what you do with your hands.

Trunk control, or trunk stability, occurs when a child has adequate stability in his trunk to maintain an upright posture, shift his weight in all directions and rotate his trunk to the left and right. Trunk control provides a base of support that allows controlled movement in the head, arms and legs.

An infant usually begins reaching for toys when his trunk is supported—either on the floor, in a supported chair or when he is held in his parent's arms. However, when the child begins to sit independently, his hands are unavailable for reaching. Those hands are busy propping him up in a sitting position. Soon, the child learns to free his hands by spreading out his legs to

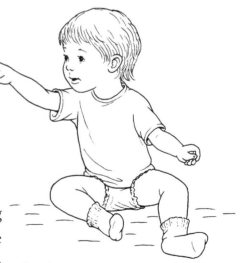

Good trunk stability allows the child to maintain balance while reaching

32

provide a wide base of support. As he gains more strength and control of the trunk, he can sit with his legs in a variety of positions. He can shift his weight and is able to turn to the left and right to reach for toys with his hands.

Trunk control is very important for developing hand skills. A child is unable to develop hand skills, especially those requiring small finger movements, if his trunk is not stable. Imagine trying to learn to knit while you are balancing on a balance beam. You need your energy to focus on more important things—like not falling off the beam! In the same way, a child needs a stable trunk to use his hands. Two things that help are strengthening the child's trunk and providing stable seating during play.

Good trunk strength and stable seating will enable your child to move yet hold himself still enough to be able to make smaller, more complex movements. A stable but active trunk will allow your child to use his hands for play and daily tasks like dressing, grooming, eating and schoolwork. So never underestimate the importance of a child's trunk in hand skills. Remember to watch your child's whole body when he is engaged in activity, and suggest that he not do his homework in the car!

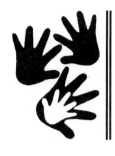

EYE WANT TO HOLD YOUR HAND

Have you ever tried to turn a lamp on in the dark? Think about what your arm and hand movements are like without your eyes to guide them. When you try to locate the lamp on the surface of the table, your movements are uncoordinated and slow. You might knock the lamp over if you aren't careful. You also will keep your hand open until you touch the lamp. Now think of turning on the lamp with other lights on in the room. With your eyes to guide you, you can easily find the lamp in the room. You don't even touch the table because the accuracy of your movements has improved. You put your hands quickly and directly on the intended goal, the lamp switch. Before you even touch the switch, you shape your hands to grasp it.

Eye-hand coordination refers to the ability of the brain to coordinate information from the eyes with the precise movements of the hand. Skillful use of the hand guided by vision is very important to human function. The activities of feeding, dressing or writing require complex eye-hand coordination. Vision gives information about an object's size, shape, texture and location. This allows you to plan the movements of your arm for the purpose of grasping the object with your hand. At the same time, the movements of your arm affect your eye movements by giving information about where the object is. What you see also allows you to plan the movements of your hand. You shape your hand according to the size and shape of the object before you even touch it. When you attempt to grasp the object, then both your eyes and hands will tell you if you were successful. Once you grasp the object, your hands will give you information about the object's size, shape, weight, temperature and texture. Your eyes and hands will continue to trade tremendous amounts of information so quickly and

EYE WANT TO HOLD YOUR HAND (continued)

smoothly that you are not even aware of it, unless something goes wrong, like knocking over a lamp when you attempt to turn on the switch.

This amazing coordination between the eyes and hand occurs very early. The newborn spends a lot of time looking at her own hands. By the time she is 6 months old, she has already begun to be able to guide her hands with her vision when reaching for a toy. The child has linked the experiences of what she is seeing with her eyes with what she is feeling with her hands. As she matures, the process of eye-hand coordination

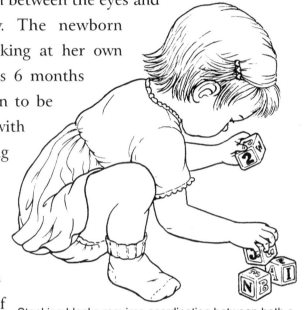

Stacking blocks requires coordination between both a child's eyes and hands.

becomes like a bridge in her brain between her eyes and her hands. After the child is 1 year old, blocks, crayons and puzzles provide opportunities to further develop this skill when using more precise movements of the hand. The child learns to imitate another person's movements in order to reproduce those same actions, such as drawing a circle. She also learns to copy objects she sees, such as making a "house" with blocks. Once the child begins school, the activities requiring eye-hand coordination become even more advanced with the demands of spelling and writing. Her eyes must be able to follow her pencil when she forms letters. The child must also have the ability to interpret what she sees on paper or a chalkboard and then duplicate it with her own hand, using a pencil.

So the next time you try to turn a lamp on in the dark, remember to pay attention to your arm and hand movements. Later, try turning on the same lamp with other lights on in the room and with your eyes to guide you. You'll probably form a new appreciation of how amazing and how important the coordination between the eyes and hands is for you and your child.

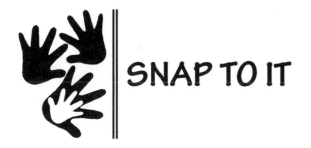

SNAP TO IT

This world would certainly be a dull place without music. What is your favorite instrumental sound? Is it the flowing song of the harp, the brassy, bold tone of the trumpet or the light whisper of the flute? To play most instruments, with only a few exceptions such as the slide trombone and some percussion pieces, the musician must move his fingers in isolation—independently from his other fingers.

Not only does isolated finger movement have a creative pursuit, it has a practical one as well. As you program your microwave to warm up a Danish or punch the numbers on your push-button telephone, observe your hand. Most likely you are poking the buttons with a straight index or pointer finger, with your other fingers tucked nicely away in your palm. This is a type of isolated finger movement that is learned because it is the most efficient position for the task. This hand position has an advantage: when you use just one finger instead of five, your touch is more precise. Also, when you activate your microwave with one finger extended and your other fingers tucked in your palm, you are better able to view the numbers on the display of the microwave.

Development of isolated finger movement begins early on. An infant first uses his whole hand, or all of his fingers together, in activities such as grasping a rattle or holding a chewing ring. Eventually, at around 6 months of age, the child's thumb begins to move independently. You can see this when the child picks up a wooden block or holds a ring in his hand. As the baby begins to creep on hands and knees or puts weight on his arms while holding a toy in his hand, he begins to develop separation of the two sides of the hand. The pinky side of the hand is on the floor helping to push the child along, while the thumb and index finger hold the toy. This is the precursor to developing individual movement of all the fingers.

The ability to poke with the index finger emerges at around 7 months of age, allowing the child to explore nooks and crevices of toys and point to pictures in a book. The next finger to develop independent movement is the pinky finger. Perhaps development occurs in this order because the easiest fingers to extend or straighten on their own are the index and pinky fingers. This is easily observed in a hand game of "Where is Thumbkin?" Tall man and ring man, the middle and ring finger respectively, are just not as willing to stand up by themselves! This can also explain

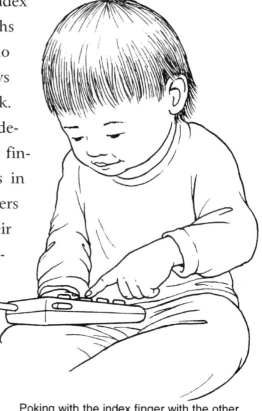

Poking with the index finger with the other fingers held in the palm

why your pinky and index finger are involved in more movement tasks on their own than your middle and ring fingers. For instance, the number of keys that the index and pinky fingers are responsible for on the standard keyboard is much more than the number of keys that the other fingers control.

As fingers learn to move independently, they also show improved skill in moving in combination with each other. You can observe this, initially, as your child becomes more proficient with using the pads of his index finger and thumb to pick up a piece of dry cereal. Later, you might observe your child making the sign "I love you" by straightening

38

his index and pinky fingers and thumb, while holding the middle and ring fingers in the palm. Or your child may rotate an object completely around in his hand, such as when turning a pencil to use the eraser. Another activity that relies on your ability to move your fingers separately is snapping. Look at your hand when you snap your fingers. Most likely, your ring and pinky fingers are held in your palm, while your middle finger presses on your thumb and then proceeds to smack into the heel of your palm to create the snapping sound. Without the ability to move your fingers independently, no sound would be produced.

So whether your child desires to become a musician or simply enjoys snapping to the beat, he will learn to appreciate the virtues of each finger's individuality!

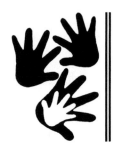

TWO SIDES OF EVERY HAND

Think of how your body responds when you catch a basketball. As the ball comes toward you, both of your arms reach symmetrically toward the ball. Your body has a center, or a midline, that your arms and legs work around. Your body also has right and left sides that work wonderfully together, but are uniquely different. Look at your hands, and you'll realize that they function in much the same way. Because of the flexible design of the bones and muscles—called arches—in your hands, your fingers and thumb all work toward the center, or midline, of your hand. Yet the two sides of the hand can also work separately, making them uniquely different.

Initially, an infant uses her ring and pinky fingers to grasp toys that are placed in her hand. Next, the child is able to use her whole hand when she grasps a toy. Around 6 months of age, the child begins to hold toys with her middle finger, index finger and thumb against her palm. When the child begins to crawl, she holds onto objects this way while putting her weight on the pinky side of the hand. This simple act begins the process of developing two markedly different sides of the hand. By 1 year old, the child is able to pick up dry cereal with her index finger and thumb while her ring finger and pinky are tucked in her palm for stability.

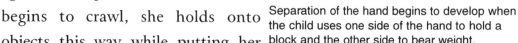

Separation of the hand begins to develop when the child uses one side of the hand to hold a block and the other side to bear weight.

Now picture yourself picking up a pencil to write your name. What position does your hand automatically take? See how your hands have two sides that work around a middle? The two sides are taking very different roles. The index finger, middle finger and thumb take the more active role of holding and moving the pencil. The ring and pinky fingers support the active side by tucking into your palm to provide stability.

We consider the more active side of the hand—the index finger, middle finger and thumb—to be the skilled side. This skilled side of the hand is responsible for highly complex and coordinated movement, such as buttoning, dialing a phone, cutting up food, turning on an egg timer or writing.

The ring and pinky fingers are less mobile and form the stability side of the hand. Although the ring and pinky fingers are not individually strong, working together they make up the powerful side of the hand. Have you ever noticed how much more difficult it is to type with your ring finger than with your index finger? The virtue of the ring and pinky fingers is in their strength, not their mobility. The stability side of the hand is responsible for the strength needed to open a screw-topped jar and is the primary part of the hand for carrying heavy objects, such as a suitcase.

If your child is having difficulty developing the two separate parts of her hand, there are different ways to encourage this skill. Have your child hold an object, such as a large ring or a small action figure, and crawl across the room. In this activity, the child will hold onto the object in the skilled side of her hand, and push off the ground using the stability side of her hand. When your child is picking up small objects, such as blocks or raisins, place a cosmetic sponge or piece of wadded-up paper in her palm and ask her to "hold it and don't let it go." This will encourage your child's ring and pinky finger to move into her palm to secure the object.

Remember that both sides of the hand can work wonderfully together and still be uniquely different. By recognizing both the differences and the strengths of each side of the hand, we are better able to understand the complexity and efficiency of our hands and how we use them. Separation of the two sides of the hand allows your child to participate in a variety of tasks, such as cutting with scissors or zipping a jacket, which require both skill and stability. Separate and conquer. Hand skills rule!

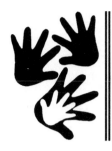

AS THE HAND TURNS

Have you noticed, now that you have a child, how good you've become at doing things with just one hand? You might have learned to hold the tube of diaper rash ointment and unscrew the lid with the same hand while holding your child down on the changing table with your other hand. You might have learned to maneuver your keys in one hand to find the car key while holding your baby on your hip with the other hand.

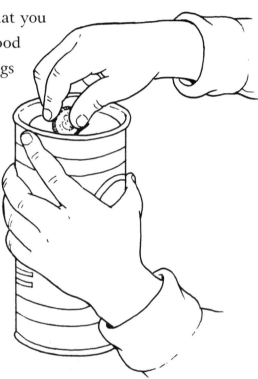

Putting money in the bank often requires moving a coin throughout the hand.

The term manipulation is used to describe movements produced by the hands in relation to an object. This ability to manipulate objects using our thumb and fingers is part of what makes humans unique. There are different ways we manipulate objects. In-hand manipulation is the ability to adjust an object in your hand to have it in a better position to use or release. Just as you learned to better adjust keys in your hand, young children learn with practice how to manipulate toys or objects in their hands.

When a baby shakes and bangs toys while holding them in her hands, she gains information about the size, shape and weight of the toys.

She'll eventually use this information to adjust her hands when she plays with a toy. When your child fingers toys, she is learning to make different movements with her individual fingers. When she holds toys in her thumb and index and ring fingers, she has learned that these fingers are more skillful in manipulating objects. She has also learned that the other side of her hand—the ring and pinky finger side—is better at providing stability for the hand. When you notice your child being able to pick up pieces of cereal and hide them in her hand or twist caps off containers, then you can be certain that her practice has paid off. These are usually the first attempts at using in-hand manipulation.

Because there are various shapes and sizes of objects, there are various ways to manipulate an object in your hand. There are three primary patterns of in-hand manipulation. The first one is translation. The name pretty much describes the pattern of movements that the hands make. When you transfer or translate a small object from your fingertips to your palm, it is appropriately called finger-to-palm translation. When you move an object in your palm to your fingertips, it is called palm-to-finger translation. You may use translation when you use a parking meter. You might pick a coin from your pocket with your fingers and then transfer it to your palm as your other hand shuts the car door. When you walk to the meter, you transfer the coin back to your fingertips to put it in the slot. If you are staying for a long time, you might put several coins in your palm and then bring one coin at a time to your fingertips to put into the machine. You may notice that your child becomes very motivated to use this pattern when candy machines are near.

Another pattern of in-hand manipulation is called shift. As the name implies, you use this pattern to shift or adjust an object to a better position for use in your hand. Typically, the object is either moved to your thumb, index finger and middle finger from the other side of your hand or it is adjusted within your thumb, index finger and middle finger. You may use shift when you write down a telephone number when calling information. You might hold a pen in your ring and pinky fingers while dialing the number. When you need to write the number down, you probably transfer the pen to your thumb and index and middle fingers to write. You also might adjust your grip on the pen so that your fingertips are closer to the writing end of the pen.

The third pattern is called rotation and is used to rotate or turn an object. Simple rotation involves turning or rolling an object between the tips of the thumb and another finger with all of them working as a unit. Complex rotation is used to turn an object in a full or half circle with the pads of the thumb and other fingers alternating their movements. You may use rotation when you add spices to your food. First you twist the bottle cap open by turning it in small increments between your fingers. You then rotate the bottle from upright to upside down to shake the spices onto your food.

In-hand manipulation is important at all stages of life, whether you are trying to get the right key on your key ring or your child is eating a handful of raisins. The ability to manipulate objects in the hand is used in a large number of activities throughout the day. This skill is needed to write with a pencil, tie shoes or eat with chopsticks. However, some of us may never learn to use chopsticks, no matter how much we practice.

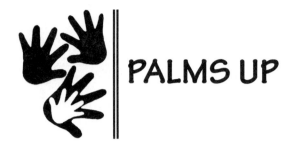

PALMS UP

Picture a child exchanging a "high 5" and "low 5" with a teammate on a soccer field. When the child's hand is positioned for the "high 5," the palm is facing away from the child's face. When the hand moves to the "low 5" position, the palm is facing up so it can be seen. In one simple hand-slapping sequence, the forearm can be observed to go from one end of its movement range—palm facing down—all the way to the other—palm facing up—in a quick and efficient movement. When the palm is down, this position is pronation. When the palm is up, this is supination. Why is the movement of the forearm important? The muscles that pronate and supinate the forearm work along with the other muscles in the arm to place the hand in the most beneficial position for the activity being performed.

The newborn's forearms are in a pronated—palms facing down—position. At 4 or 5 months, when the child begins to take weight onto his forearms as he lies on his tummy, the muscles that pronate the arm are slowly stretched. This stretching allows for more supination—palms facing up—positioning to occur. The muscles of the forearm, both those that pronate and supinate the arm, are strengthened as the baby moves over his arms from side to side to reach for a toy. At around 9 months of age, when he can sit with a steady trunk, the baby is able to fully supinate the arm. This allows him to turn an object over to explore the other side. In the next few months, as refinement of fine motor skills continues, you begin to see a slight forearm supination in conjunction with better use of the thumb, index and middle finger, what we call the skilled side of the hand. You will see the child use slight forearm supination to pick up dry cereal with his fingertips. This position allows for a better view of the object in the fingertips.

PALMS UP (continued)

Both positions of the forearm have their advantages. When you are working with a pronated forearm—palm facing down—you are most likely working on a surface. You could be wiping off a chalkboard, holding a tomato in order to cut it or keeping a piece of paper steady while you write. Working on a surface allows you to put more power into the activity. On the other hand, when you are working with a supinated forearm—palm facing up—you are better able to visually focus on the object. Picture how you might view a ladybug in your hand or hold a book to read.

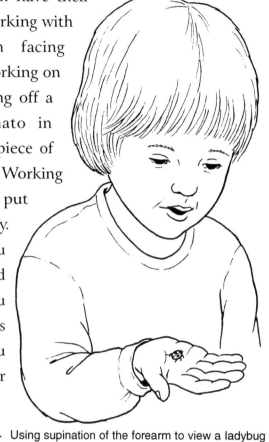

Using supination of the forearm to view a ladybug

Most of the time, though, our forearms are neither fully pronated nor fully supinated. They are somewhere in between. You can see this when you hammer a nail, hold onto ropes on a swing or use a pencil to draw.

It is interesting that most hygiene and self-care tasks from the tummy down on the front side of the body, such as zipping pants, painting toenails or tying shoes, involve more pronation—palm facing down. Activities from the chest up and on the back side of the body, such as putting on earrings, eating or brushing your hair, involve more supination—palm facing up. These differences occur because of where the activity takes place.

Because the muscles that supinate the arm are strengthened later than the muscles that pronate the arm in a child's development, a child who is challenged in a new activity might attempt to stabilize his forearm by holding it in a fully pronated position. This position has been historically stronger for him. For instance, a child who is just learning to cut paper with scissors may fully pronate his forearm while cutting. This can easily be identified by a child's appearance of cutting sideways down the paper instead of cutting straight across.

Both positions of the forearm, and combinations of these positions, are important for different reasons and different activities. By paying attention to how your child positions his arm for various tasks, you can be a better observer and a better teacher. All right—give me five!

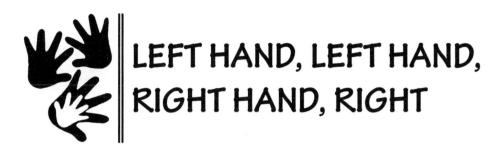

LEFT HAND, LEFT HAND, RIGHT HAND, RIGHT

As parents, we often wonder how our child will develop. Will she look like mom or dad? Will she be tall or short? What will her personality be like? Many parents are also curious about whether their child is going to be left- or right-handed. Have you ever watched closely which hand your child uses? Have you tried to recall which hand each relative uses? If so,

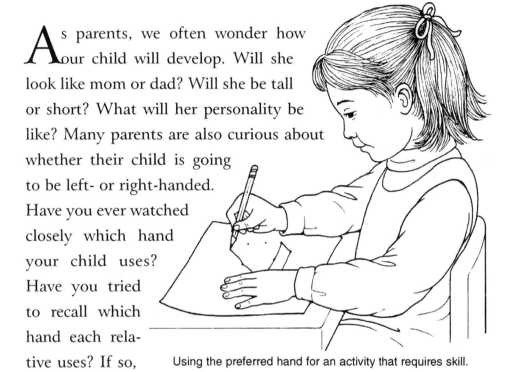

Using the preferred hand for an activity that requires skill.

then you may be interested in knowing something about handedness.

Although there are some subtle indicators of hand preference that can be observed in young infants, you should be concerned if your child uses one hand more than the other before she is 18 months old. You should also be aware that there is still debate among experts about when a preference for one hand should emerge. Yet, there are some general guidelines to consider. The very earliest that you can observe a clear preference is around 3 to 4 years. However, many typical 3-year-olds use either hand interchangeably, at times appearing to prefer one hand and then, later, the other.

Hand dominance is the definitive use of one hand. It appears to correlate with the development of a mature pencil grasp. Hand dominance is usually not seen until age 4, and sometimes as late as 6 years of age. A strongly established dominance may not even occur until 8 or 9 years of age. Some individuals remain, to some extent, ambidextrous their whole lives. A child may use either hand, no matter what the task, or she may use a specific hand for certain tasks. For example, she may use the right hand for writing but the left for throwing a ball.

Handedness refers to which hand the child uses in activities that require only one hand as well as what role each hand takes in activities that require both hands. In two-handed activities, the preferred hand leads while the other hand assists. The reasons why individuals choose to use the left or right hand exclusively or both hands interchangeably are not always obvious. Heredity appears often, but not always, to be the reason for handedness. There is a greater incidence of left-handedness in children with one or both parents who are left-handed.

When attempting to determine your child's handedness, consider that people use different hands for different tasks. Activities such as coloring, cutting or stringing require the skills of the preferred hand. However, activities such as pushing a door open, picking up a large ball or pulling a wagon do not require the use of the preferred hand. In these situations, the child may use whatever hand is convenient or available. Whether or not the task is familiar also determines which hand the child will use. If the child must plan her movements, then she will tend to use the more skilled hand to be successful in the new task. Factors such as the size, shape, weight and location of the object may also determine which hand she uses.

It is best to not insist your child use a certain hand. In the past, professionals pushed children to use their right hand for writing. However, we now realize that this approach can actually cause more problems for a child learning to write. Now, many experts believe that

LEFT HAND, LEFT HAND, RIGHT HAND, RIGHT
(continued)

by the age of 8 years, a child should be encouraged to develop proficiency in one hand, whether right or left. Yet, even this philosophy is being questioned. It is true that a lack of hand preference can be an indicator of learning disabilities. However, it is usually only one of many symptoms, such as clumsiness or problems in school. In fact, there are many people who are ambidextrous who successfully use both hands interchangeably.

So, it's fun to guess what hand your child will use, but it's best to let your child make the choice. As you can see, handedness, like so many other characteristics, can develop very differently in each child. That's what makes our children unique and our lives as parents interesting.

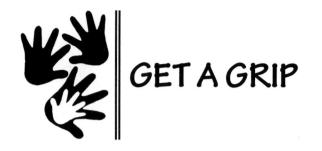

GET A GRIP

When you think about using your hands with objects, which one of these things is not like the others: a suitcase, a baseball, a feather and a jar of peanut butter? Give up? Maybe you've guessed because of the title of the article. If you picked a feather, you were right. The feather requires a precision grasp and the others require a power grasp. What's the difference? With a precision grasp, you typically hold an object between your thumb and fingertips. The object is usually small. Just like its name, with a power grasp, you typically exert force or power on an object with your fingers and thumb acting against the palm of your hand. You've experienced someone else's power grasp if your hand has ever hurt after shaking hands with someone. Usually a power grasp is used for medium or large objects, like when you open a door using a doorknob or when you lift a piece of furniture.

Because objects come in various shapes, you need various power grasps to handle them. There are three different types of power grasps. One kind of grasp is called the hook grasp, which looks and functions a lot like its name. When you use it, you bend all or most of the joints of your fingers, except the thumb, to create a hook. You use the hook grasp when you need strength to carry an object like a heavy suitcase.

Another power grasp is the cylindric grasp, whose name implies the cylindrical shape of the objects for which it is used. When you use this grasp, your fingers are close together and bent to wrap around the object. Your thumb is usually wrapped around the other side of the object, in opposition. All or part of your palm is in contact with the object. How much the object is in contact with your palm usually

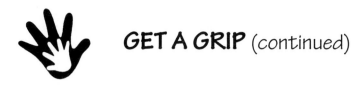

depends on the how much force you are exerting on the object or the size or weight of the object. For example, you may hold a full can of soda tighter in your palm than an empty one. You also use this grasp when you wring a wet beach towel or hold a rolled-up magazine to swat a fly.

The other grasp is the spheric grasp, which, as the name hints, is used to hold spherical or round objects. With this grasp, your fingers are spread apart and bent with all, part or none of your palm in contact with the object. As with the cylindrical grasp, how much the object is in contact with your palm depends on the how much force you exert on the object or the size or weight of the object. You use this grasp for objects like tennis balls or when you try to open a large jar of pickles.

When your child holds his spoon or crayon in his whole hand in the first few years of life, that is not to be mistaken for a power grasp. That grasp is an early and temporary grasp that is used before a more mature grasp is developed. When your 5-year-old is gripping onto the spoon with all his might to dig hard ice cream out of the carton, that is a power grasp.

So when you see your child pulling a wagon by the handle, you'll know he is using a power grasp called a hook grasp. When he pulls pop beads apart, you'll know that he is using a cylindrical grasp. And, when you see your child remove the lid from a jar of lightning bugs, you'll know he's using a spherical grasp. But, you'll also know when your child picks up a small bird feather with his fingertips and thumb, he is using a precision grasp and not a power grasp.

Using a spheric grasp to open a jar

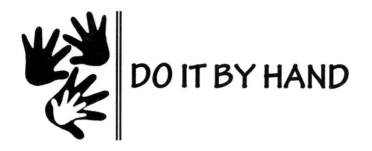

DO IT BY HAND

As adults, we rarely face tasks in our daily routine that are so difficult that we have to stop and think about how we are going to do them. Imagine if you had to think through every step of brushing your teeth or making your bed. Your mental energy would be spent before you even started the day. There are situations in life when we do have to think about a task and plan our movements. Usually these are new and unfamiliar situations. Have you ever gone to an aerobics or karate class where you were tripping over your own feet trying to follow the teacher's moves? Learning a new sport like karate, or a new hobby like knitting, can be exhausting and almost stressful because you have to think about every move. What is going on in these circumstances? It's probably not that you don't have the ability to kick or jump. You have to use your skill of motor planning much more than you do with a task you are accustomed to. As you learn new skills, you have to take all the information from your different senses to plan and carry out your movements. In an aerobics class, for example, your movements must correspond with what you hear—the beat of the music and the instructions of the teacher—and what you see—the teacher's dance routine.

So what is motor planning? It is the ability to interact with things in the world around you in a purposeful way based on the information you perceive. This means being able to have the idea of what to do with something, plan how to do it and then carry out the plan. It is the bridge between intellect and doing. Think of how many purposeful tasks you do with your hands. You eat, dress, write, type on the computer, play board games and more. So, the ability to plan our hand movements has a profound effect on our daily activities. This is the

Reproducible. © 2001 by PRO-ED, Inc.
Handprints–Pieraccini and Vance

same for your child. In fact, so many daily tasks and objects are new and unfamiliar to a child that his ability to motor plan hand movements is constantly being challenged.

In the first year of life, a child explores toys and objects with his senses, feeling them with his hands and mouth and inspecting them with his eyes. As the young child learns about characteristics of objects, such as toys, he begins to experiment with how best to use them. Once he learns the best way to use a toy, he may repeat the action over and over to reinforce what he has learned. For example, a child may delight in repeatedly hitting the lever on a toy for it to make music. This repetition allows the child to create memories of the relationship between his movements and his sensory experiences.

By 2 years old, a child should know how to play with a wide variety of age-appropriate toys. The ability to motor plan initially becomes evident in the purposefulness of the child's play. Although spontaneous, a child's play should have intent and an organized approach. The child may know that he can line up blocks, stack them, put them in a container and

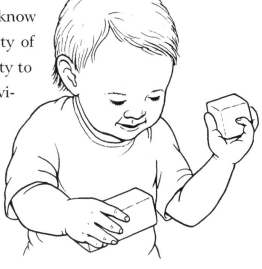

Handling different shaped blocks requires motor planning skills

much more. If he plays with blocks that are cube-shaped, but goes to a friend's house who has rectangular or cylindrical blocks, he probably will still have an idea of what to do with these toys based on previous experiences. However, he may have to plan his movements to manipulate blocks with different shapes. A child who has difficulty with motor planning may not know what to do with the blocks. He may just stare at the blocks and not attempt to construct anything. Sometimes a child will choose to scatter or throw the blocks to avoid the task. The child who has an idea of what to do with the blocks but does not know how to plan his movements may place each block in a different place on the table but not put them together to create anything. If the child has increasing success interacting with objects in his environment, he will develop a storehouse of memories of what movements are reliable to use to perform familiar tasks. The child will remember how to hold and place the blocks to stack them. These memories allow many tasks to become more automatic and, consequently, require less focus and thought. This storehouse of movements can also be used as a reference for new tasks. Although the child may have to hold and place the blocks differently, he still will be able to stack blocks that are shaped differently from his own blocks.

As children grow older, many new activities require more skill and, therefore, more complex motor planning. For many tasks, whether in play, self-help or academics, the planning process requires not just one but a series of movements to make up one total and smooth action. This need to sequence hand movements can be seen in handwriting or tying shoelaces. When a child enters school, the ability to motor plan directly affects his success in many areas. Many activities in gym class, such as a game of dodge ball, require instantaneous motor planning. A child does not have much time to decide whether to catch or dodge a ball when it is coming straight at him. Writing requires a child to be able to copy someone else's movements to form letters. Then he needs to develop a consistent way to make each letter so he does not hesitate before writing each letter in a word. He must have a consistent way to hold a pencil. If he uses a different grasp every time, he won't be able to experience how it feels to make each letter.

DO IT BY HAND (continued)

So, though we may laugh at ourselves when we trip over our own feet in an aerobics class, motor planning is a crucial skill we need to perform all of life's tasks. The ability to motor plan allows your child to make his own mark on the world around him.

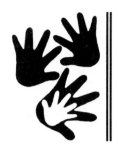

KEEP AN EYE ON IT

If you have ever driven down a curvy road in an unfamiliar area at night, you might recall being thankful for the road signs with arrows and lines making you aware of the road changes up ahead. Your eyes perceive which direction the arrow is pointing and then your muscles react by braking and turning the wheel accordingly. What you perceive, or your visual perception in this case, affects your ability to move in an accurate, efficient and timely manner.

There are many different ways your eyes can perceive information that helps you better understand, distinguish, compare or remember what you see. Your eyes help you find that jigsaw puzzle piece with part of a blue roof on it among the rest of the pieces. Your eyes help you locate your child's favorite book when it is hiding halfway under the bed or when it is turned upside down. Your eyes tell you how far you must reach to pick up a glass of tea. Your eyes can pick out the difference between a "b" and a "d" and give you the information you need to create a space between written words. Your eyes even play a role in helping you remember what something looked like, such as recalling a telephone number or a word in a crossword puzzle.

It is important to note that visual acuity is a different skill than visual perception. Clear and accurate vision is vital, but it is different from understanding what you are seeing. Memory also plays a role in visual perception. If you can recall what a letter looked like on the chalkboard, you will be more successful when writing it on your paper.

Interestingly, an infant uses hand skills to help him develop the ability to perceive things with his eyes through grasping, poking and manipulating objects. By learning about concepts such as hard, soft,

58

flat, curved, same and different with his hands, the child is teaching his eyes to perceive these concepts as well. When your child advances from placing shapes into a shape sorter using the trial-and-error method, in which he tests each piece in each spot, to placing the shapes successfully on the first attempt, you know that he is beginning to perceive same and different with his eyes. Eventually, his hands rely on what his eyes perceive to assist him with more complex hand movements, such as knowing which side of the shirt is the outside when he is putting it on or being able to use a crayon to copy a shape or letter.

So as you can see, a child's ability to perceive information with his eyes directly affects his hand skills in tasks requiring communication between the eyes and hands, such as copying a block design or learning how to print. Often, it is hard to determine whether the child is having problems with how his eyes perceive information or how this information is then processed and communicated from his eyes to his hands. For example, is it difficult for him to pick out which triangle is different, or is the problem that he cannot accurately draw a triangle? If your child is having difficulty imitating letters or designs, he can be tested to determine whether his problem is with what he is perceiving with his eyes or with the connection between his eyes and his hands.

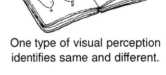

One type of visual perception identifies same and different.

It is important to note that we all perceive things differently, as when two children are looking at the same cloud and one sees an elephant and the other sees a mouse. These differences are part of what makes us unique and special as we journey through our lives. Even so, we want to make sure that we can all read the map or road signs on the way.

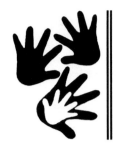

STAYING IN TOUCH

Many of us have played the game at a party where you have to identify common objects like coins or paper clips in a bag without looking. Were you the one who identified the most or least items? If you haven't played this game, then you probably have searched through a pocket or purse for money or keys without looking. This abili-

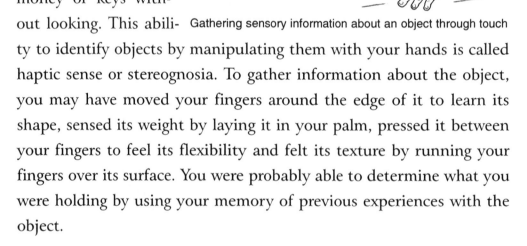

Gathering sensory information about an object through touch

ty to identify objects by manipulating them with your hands is called haptic sense or stereognosia. To gather information about the object, you may have moved your fingers around the edge of it to learn its shape, sensed its weight by laying it in your palm, pressed it between your fingers to feel its flexibility and felt its texture by running your fingers over its surface. You were probably able to determine what you were holding by using your memory of previous experiences with the object.

Do you know what allows you to do this with your hands? There are several structures present in the hand and all parts of the body that send sensory information about an object to the brain. These structures, called nerve receptors, are very numerous and dense in the hand. One set of receptors that provides information about how the object feels is found in the fat pads and ridges in your hand. Another set is found in the muscles of the hand. This set also provides information about how the object feels and the position of the hand as it

60

manipulates the object. A third set of receptors in the tendons of a muscle senses the tension of the muscle. These receptors sense the force required to handle an object. One last set detects the movement in the joints of the hand, including the direction and rate of movement. All of the information gathered by these receptors allows you to identify an object without the help of your eyes or other senses.

Typically, though, your vision and your haptic sense work together to help you gather information about objects in your daily life. If you are unable to feel the quarter you are sure you have in the change pocket of your wallet, you will probably look briefly so that you can place your finger in the right location to retrieve the coin.

You develop this skill of haptic sense as an infant. Initially, an infant uses both hands and his mouth to learn about the characteristics of an object. This is not always a toy; all of us have probably been amazed at the flexibility of a baby who takes his foot into his mouth. By 6 months of age, a child is beginning to combine information about an object by using his eyes, his hands and his mouth. This allows the child to begin to associate stuffed animals with softness, for example. Although much is not known about the development of haptic sense, we do know that by the age of 2½, children can begin to identify many familiar objects with their hands while their vision is blocked. Around 4 years of age, they often can identify shapes, such as squares or circles, through touch alone. As children mature, these skills continue to become more sophisticated. Increased sensitivity of the hands allows a child to distinguish between textures of objects. For example, a 7-year-old can probably feel his favorite sweatshirt buried under other clothing in a gym bag. Improved ability to methodically probe objects also helps a child tell if an object is turned or facing up or down. So, if a brush were also buried in the bag, the child could identify if the brush or the handle end were upright.

STAYING IN TOUCH (continued)

The ability to manipulate objects without relying on your other senses is not just necessary for finding coins. You often button a shirt or tie shoes without looking. You depend on your haptic sense to hook the clasp of a necklace or put a rubber band in your hair for a ponytail. Throughout your daily routine, you rely on this sense to identify objects, or parts of objects, to complete all the necessary tasks.

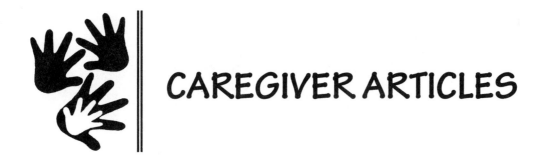

CAREGIVER ARTICLES

HAND SKILLS IN DAILY ACTIVITIES

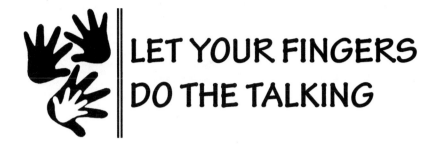

LET YOUR FINGERS DO THE TALKING

Have you ever tried to talk to someone in a foreign language of which you only knew a few words? It can be a very frustrating experience. Those few words were probably not adequate for all that you wanted to say. A child who has few or no words can feel the same frustration about not being able to communicate needs and wants. You can avoid this frustration by introducing sign language, not only to children with hearing impairments, but to all children. A child usually develops the skills to make gestures with his hands before he can produce words. Sign language can serve as a temporary or a permanent bridge to verbal communication.

There are many benefits for a child to learn sign language. It decreases frustration and in so doing may keep the child from whining or having outbursts. There is also proof that it accelerates a child's learning to talk, improves intelligence, promotes social skills and encourages early opportunities for bonding between the child and parent.

So what is sign language? Sign language uses gestures of the hands, often in relation to the body, to communicate with others. Some babies have learned signs as early as 8 months old. How easily a child learns the gestures for signs depends primarily on how mature his hand skills are. Two common first signs for young children are "more" and "eat." The sign "more" is displayed by having the hands touch at the fingertips in front of the chest. The sign for "eat" consists of one hand, with fingers brought together, moving towards the mouth.

Besides the obvious reason that these two signs have important meaning to a young child, why are they and others like them favorite firsts? They require only the skills that the child's hands have already mastered.

The signs for "more" and "eat" require movement only from the shoulder and the elbow with the hands being still. A child develops control of his trunk first, and then he slowly gains control of movement down the arm so that the shoulder and elbow are controlled before the hand. Therefore, signs that require movement of the hand are more difficult. These movements are also large, with very little coordination required. As you probably know, beginning movement is often very uncoordinated.

Signing the word "more"

A baby learns to grasp objects close to his body before he can reach for objects far away. The signs for "more" and "eat" both bring the hands toward the center of the body. The sign for "eat" even brings the hand toward the mouth, a movement that has been refined by the mouthing of toys. Hand movements that move away from the body are harder. Both signs allow body parts to touch, giving the child feedback about the accuracy of his hand movements. It's harder to make movement in mid-air. That may be one reason that many children learn to clap their hands before they can wave. Both signs are performed in front of the eyes where the child can tell if his movements are accurate. Even for adults, it's hard to do a new hand skill without looking.

As a child's hand skills develop, his repertoire of signs will continue to expand. One-handed signs or signs where the hands do the same thing

LET YOUR FINGERS DO THE TALKING (continued)

are easier. The child does not have to coordinate movement of both sides of his body as much as he would if his hands had to do two different movements. However, as a child begins to develop hand dominance, he can increasingly do tasks, such as stringing beads, where the hands do different movements. As the child learns to use his fingers separately, such as when snapping his fingers, he can then learn finger spelling. Finger spelling uses 26 hand positions that represent the letters of the alphabet.

As your child learns sign language, be aware that his gestures do not have to be exact. It is okay for children to even make up their own signs if it is easier for them. This allows them to have more signs before their hand skills develop. In fact, many experts recommend making up simpler signs instead of signs used by the American Sign Language (ASL) method. Gestures that require less mature hand skills and that are symbolically more like the object being signed are easier. For example, it is easy for a child to gesture "airplane" by holding both arms out to his sides at shoulder level. It would be more difficult for him to make the ASL sign for airplane by holding his hand away from his body with some fingers straight and some bent.

It is also important to know that gestures do the job of words, but it is incorrect to think that gestures always replace words, even in standard sign language. The gestures can represent concepts, just as words do. However, just as the gestures are dependent on the development of hand skills, the ability to understand symbols and concepts is dependent on the development of language skills. So it's okay if your child initially signs "cracker" when you pull the cookie box out of the cupboard, but your child should eventually learn to sign the word "cookie."

Although children's skills for sign language come sooner than those for speech, you still need patience and consistency to teach them to your

67

child. Just remember how you may have first struggled to communicate to someone in a foreign language. Was it hard to shape your mouth to make the sounds for the first time? Was it hard to remember what the words were? Your child is going through a similar process as he learns to communicate, whether he's using sign language or speech.

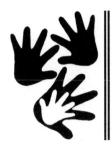

RAISE A GLASS

Think back to the last soda commercial you saw. When the actor took a big swig of cola, did you even think about his hands? Probably not, in the same way that you don't consciously think about your own hands when you are drinking. This skill has become automatic because you started learning it way back in the first half of the first year of your life!

Hand skills can affect a child's ability to drink independently. Before the age of 6 months, an infant is fed liquids generally by the breast or the bottle. Initially, a child ori-

Early drinking from a cup using two hands

ents to a breast or the bottle in response to a touch on the cheek. Eye-hand coordination begins later, when the child is able to locate a bottle or breast with his eyes and can reach his hands toward the object.

Initially, a child will suck his fingers when they are close to his mouth. As the child begins bringing his hands or toys to his mouth, he is developing the beginning skills for hand-to-mouth patterns used later in drinking. A child will start to pat the bottle with one or both hands and this will quickly develop into holding the bottle himself, which occurs in the last half of the child's first year. By 10 months of age, the controlled movement of the child's arms and hands allows him to use both hands together to bring a bottle to his mouth and tip it adequately so he can drink.

When the child has adequate control of his head and trunk to sit unsupported, he can be introduced to drinking from an open cup held by an adult. You can assist your child by holding the cup while he guides it. Around his first year, he will be able to hold a cup using his two hands pressed on the side of the cup and drink by himself, with much spilling. During the transition from bottle to cup, parents will often use covered sipping or spouted cups because the child has not yet understood the difference between bringing the bottle to his mouth as opposed to the open cup. At this time, a child will often rest his elbows on his high-chair tray or the sides of his body to support his arm movements. At around a year and a half, he will be able to use the pads of his fingers and thumb to secure and tilt the cup for drinking with slightly less spilling. However, not until he is 2 years old will he be able to drink with minimal spilling from a cup. Initially, the child will drink from the cup with two hands, but soon he will attempt to hold the cup with one hand while the other hand waits nearby to help if needed. As this skill is practiced, the child will be able to drink without spilling using only one hand some time in his third year.

If your child does have difficulty with the hand skills needed to drink on his own, there are a few adaptations that might allow him to be more independent. Using a cup with handles can help your child hold onto his cup with a tightly fisted hand as opposed to the shallow cupping of the hand needed to hold a cup without handles. A straw placed in the cup can also be used to eliminate hand use altogether.

So as you sit back in your comfy chair and take your own swig of cola, appreciate the "behind the scenes" work of your hands. Recognizing the importance of the hands allows you to be a better observer and teacher as your child goes through the process of learning to drink. So raise your glass! Here's to parenting!

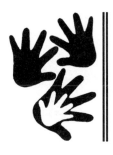

GRAB A BITE TO EAT

Every step of independence your child takes is really a step toward freedom for you. Although we want to cherish every stage of our children's growing up, it is nice when they are able to feed themselves. Don't you find it hard to savor a meal when you are alternating bites of food from your plate for yourself with spoonfuls of baby food for your child?

Your child needs to acquire many skills before he is truly able to feed himself. Coordination between the eyes and hands for feeding or drinking begins when he is able to locate a bottle or breast with his eyes. When he begins taking his hands or toys to his mouth, he is also developing hand-to-mouth patterns for independent feeding. By 10 months of age, a child typically can bring a bottle to his mouth with his hands, which is the first step to independence!

A child may first attempt finger feeding by holding a cracker with his whole hand and smashing it into his mouth with his palm. This often results in just as much cracker on the child's face as in his mouth. Initially, a young child may not have the ability to grasp the food with the appropriate amount of pressure, so crackers are often broken in the hand. As he acquires more advanced

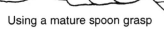
Using a mature spoon grasp

skills, however, the young child is able to feed himself dry cereal, crackers and small pieces of soft fruit or vegetables.

A child's finger feeding becomes more advanced as he learns to use a pincer grasp, using the thumb and index fingers, and as he learns to control the movements of his arms. The child must also be able to hold his jaw steady enough to place the food inside his mouth while using a pincer grasp. Otherwise, he might drop the food back into his palm and push it into the mouth.

At approximately 18 months of age, utensil use emerges with the use of a cup and spoon. Your child may be interested in using a spoon before this. He will probably enjoy holding, stirring or banging with the spoon, but he will be unable to fill the spoon with food. If he is successful in securing food on the spoon, he will often

More advanced finger feeding uses a pincer grasp.

turn the spoon upside down before it reaches his mouth. When he is finally successful in taking the food to his mouth, much spilling occurs because of his inability to control his arm and hand movements. To feed himself with a spoon, the child must be able to maintain a raised arm and adjust the movements of the arm to move the spoon through space. Usually the ability to use a spoon and cup without spilling emerge at the same time.

By 3 years of age, a child probably has learned to successfully use a fork to spear pieces of food. The common method used at this age is to stab the food and shovel it to the mouth. The 3-year-old does not have the advanced hand skills needed for the refined use of a fork. He must develop a more mature grasp that uses the fingers to hold the fork and good eye-hand coordination to stab small pieces of food. It is not until middle childhood that the child's tool use is advanced enough to use a butter knife well.

So the process of gaining independence and freedom is a long road for you and your child. There are many bumps along the road, such as those stains that won't come out of that sweet dress you splurged on or the battle with the mess on the floor under the kitchen table. Or the pieces of rotting food you find in odd places in the house. Yet, each bump is also a step forward toward independence.

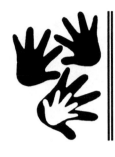

ONE, TWO, BUCKLE MY SHOE

Dressing is complex. That statement may sound silly to you because you have been dressing yourself for so long that you are on autopilot. This allows you to be engaged in other activities such as talking on the phone, putting on makeup or listening to a favorite radio program while you are dressing. Your child may be able to do this, too, but only after a great deal of practicing the skill. When your child starts telling you a story while she puts on her clothes, you'll know that she has mastered the skill of dressing.

Dressing involves a complex set of skills that is slowly developed and refined over a long period of time. A child will first "participate" in dressing when she pulls at her clothes at 3 months of age. Eventually a child can learn how to tie a man's tie at approximately 10 years of age.

Dressing involves a number of separate skills used together to complete the task. One skill is the child's ability to take in information with her eyes, such as visually locating the heel of the sock. Another skill involves the child's ability to plan movements, such as visualizing how to pull the sock over her toes. Finally, the child needs to be able to carry out these movements using both large and small muscles, such as bending down and using two hands to put on and pull up the sock.

As your child's hand skills improve, so does her ability to undress and dress herself. Ironically, undressing comes before dressing. So just as soon as you have clothed your child, she will be able to successfully pull everything off. She won't, however, be able to dress herself again. This occurs because undressing uses primitive hand skills, such as using a whole hand to grasp, that allow the child to pull or push off her clothes. In fact, a child can often remove clothes using just one hand. Putting clothes on, however, often requires the use of two hands together, which is a skill that comes later. Also, undressing requires simpler visual-perceptual skills. It doesn't matter which side is the front or the back when it's coming off! A child haphazardly begins pulling off items of clothing such as socks or a hat in the first year of life. Clothes come off in a more meaningful fashion at around a year and a half. As the child learns to use both hands together, she can do more sophisticated undressing, such as removing underpants and pants around her second year or removing a T-shirt later in her second year.

The next major stepping stone for the child is being able to dress herself in clothes without fasteners. At this point, the child has established better use of both hands together, as well as a strong power grasp. She can pull up a pair of socks or pants around the third year, or a pullover garment later in the third year. Generally, putting clothes on your legs and feet tends to be easier than putting garments on your arms and trunk. Therefore, we can expect that the child will be able to put on her pants and socks before she can put on shirts or dresses. Near the end of the fifth year, a child becomes proficient in turning clothes the correct way and putting shoes on the correct foot.

As her hand skills mature, the child begins to use more refined movements. She can use her fingertips together with good strength, moving objects in her hand and using both hands together as a team. At this point, the child is ready to meet the challenge of managing fasteners on clothing or jewelry. In this stage of development, her ability to visually understand what she is looking at is very important. In order to orient the button with the hole or figure out the sequence for shoe tying, the eyes must correctly convey information to the brain so it can guide the hands to the right place. As with undressing and then dressing, opening fasteners typically precedes closing them. As expected, success with fasteners located at the front and middle of the body, such as buttons on a vest or snaps on a shirt, comes before success with fasteners that are harder to reach and see. Zippers on the back of a shirt or buttons on a side pocket are harder for the child to reach and see. Success with fasteners in these positions will develop later. The zipper is often the first fastener the child can successfully manipulate at around the second year, followed by large buttons during the latter half of the second year. With practice, the child will become more

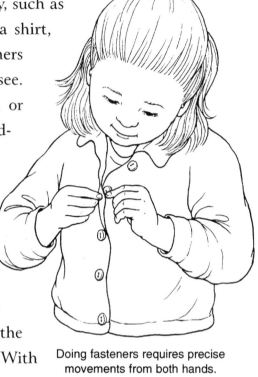

Doing fasteners requires precise movements from both hands.

proficient using her eyes and hands together. This will allow her to buckle her belt or shoes around the fourth year and tie her shoes around the sixth year. It takes even more practice at these skills before the child can work buttons, ties or clasps without using her eyes to guide her, as when she buttons a top back button or puts on a necklace.

An important thing to consider when teaching your child to dress is the type of clothing she wears. If you provide loose-fitting clothes with large head openings and pants with elastic waistlines, your child can be more successful in early dressing than if she has tight clothes with many fasteners. Encourage your child to practice these skills through dress-up play with your old clothes, which tend to be larger. If you want to start working on fasteners with your child, purchase clothes with larger buttons placed in the middle of the garment. Or get clothes with soft snaps that do not require excessive force. This will allow your child to be independent with fasteners more quickly.

As you can see, dressing is complex. So when your child appears—shirt on inside-out and backward—with a grin on her face, and says, "Look what I did!" you can truly appreciate just what an accomplishment this really is!

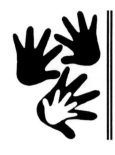

COME OUT AND PLAY WITH ME

Children can spend hours and hours in play. As adults, we may be tempted to think their activity is without purpose, but play could be considered a child's work. Play is how a child learns about the world around him. During play, the child develops and masters skills that are the building blocks for the rest of life. Toys and household objects are the tools he uses. The young child who loves to play in the kitchen cabinet where the pots and pans are stored is getting an opportunity to learn about different weights, sizes, textures and shapes of various objects and how all these objects relate to each other. The child is also developing coordination between his hands and eyes and discovering how many ways he can manipulate each container. He may learn about the pots and pans by banging on them; putting toys in them; stacking, nesting and knocking them down. Then he'll move on to the Tupperware® cabinet to repeat the same process.

A baby typically learns about the characteristics of a toy by feeling it with his hands while exploring it with his eyes. You may notice that, initially, a baby's play is very repetitive. These repetitive interactions allow him to learn not only about the object, but how to handle it. You may see your child use his hands to bang, shake, scratch or swat at toys. Initially, a baby will handle all toys in the same way despite each object's different attributes or uses. However, as the child learns that there are differences in toys, he may decide to shake the rattle that makes noise but scratch at the book with different textures. Although the child's handling of toys is very simple, this is the first stage of play. This play is both purposeful and done for enjoyment.

By a child's first birthday, he has learned about the qualities and uses of many different objects. He also has increased control of his hands to better manipulate these objects. He may use his two hands together by holding a toy with one hand while he explores it with the other. The child may also have learned that to hold a bottle requires both hands, but a piece of cereal is easier to hold with one hand using the tips of his thumb and index finger. Also, the child has begun to use two or more toys together—like banging pots and pans together. And, although you may be driven to distraction, your child's ability to manipulate objects and coordinate his eyes and hands is being perfected with each crash. During play, the child will continue to test and verify the information he has learned about objects by repeatedly returning to the same activity. He enjoys the predictability of seeing the little animal pop up when he pulls the lever on the toy. After the first birthday play is used to further understand how objects can be used, particularly how different objects or parts of objects relate to each other. The child begins to stack blocks, turn pages of storybooks and open and shut lids of containers.

When a child turns 2 years old, the information gained by exploring toys and objects through play is put to good use. He will be able to look at a toy, form an idea of how to use it and interact with it based on previous experiences. At first, the child is more successful with toys that have obvious uses. By preschool, though, the child can use materials that lack shape and form, such as play dough, to create something with his hands that he has visualized in his mind. This requires very sophisticated skills of remembering what the object looks like and then being able to manipulate the material with his hands to create what is intended.

Another type of play also emerges around 2 years old which many people call imaginary play. Imaginary play is not limited by the objects or people available, nor restricted by time and place. At first, a child may imitate what he frequently sees the adults around him do. His play usually relates the objects to himself. For example, he may pretend to brush his teeth or comb his hair by shaping his hands as if holding the object. Later, he may incorporate dolls, stuffed animals, figurines or other people into his play. This is a great opportunity for the child to refine his hand skills for self-help such as feeding or dressing. He can pretend to feed a doll with a bottle or a spoon or dress the doll.

During the child's preschool years, hand skills take an increasingly important role in play. Art projects that use cutting, coloring or gluing require the child to have very complex hand coordination. Puzzles with 12 or more interconnected pieces require coordinated use of the eyes and hands. Pouring imaginary tea from a teapot into a teacup also requires good coordination between the hands. Overall, what appears to be ordinary play is actually a powerful instrument for a child to learn about his world. Play allows

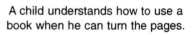

A child understands how to use a book when he can turn the pages.

the child to gain competence and, consequently, confidence in his hand skills as well as in many other areas of life. Adults can only wish that all the important things of life could be so enjoyable.

Reproducible. © 2001 by PRO-ED, Inc.
Handprints–Pieraccini and Vance

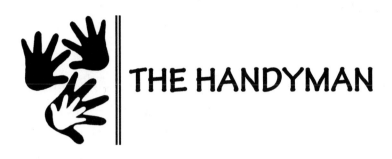

THE HANDYMAN

Have you noticed that it's difficult to write a letter or fill out a form within reach of a toddler? He is fascinated with the pen and can be quite persistent in trying to get it from you. Some of us have learned the hard way by accidentally leaving a pen and important papers out. All you need is one bad experience to realize that children love to imitate adults using tools. In the toy stores, there are toy hammers already in the baby section. By the time you move to the pre-school section, there are kits with kitchen utensils and home repair tools that are probably more complete than what you have in your kitchen and garage. Tools used by young children are not limited to toys. Items like spoons, forks and hairbrushes are also part of your child's toolbox. The variety of tools you use expands throughout life. In an adult's life, the use of tools can include ski poles, a broom or gardening shears. You use tools as an extension of your arms to allow you to perform a task better than you could with just your hands. Without a broom or a vacuum, you would have to pick up every piece of dirt from your floor by hand.

There are several skills your child should master before you introduce the use of tools, such as a spoon. The child must have the ability to maintain his balance while sitting so his hands are free to use the utensil. He needs the basic skills of reach, grasp and release to handle the utensil. The child also must have adequate attention so he can watch his parents model the correct use of the tool.

The child's beginning attempts with a tool will be crude. For example, using a spoon will probably result in more food on the table than in his mouth, but like any other skill, practice will make perfect. As the child's hand skills develop—as he learns to better manipulate objects, coordinate his eyes and hands and use his hands together—his use of tools will continue to improve. It may take several years, though, for the child to acquire the ability to use more advanced tools such as ski poles.

Although a child may initially try a variety of grasps when using a tool, he eventually learns what grasp works best with a certain tool and then continues to use that grasp. With a pencil, he must use a grasp that allows for precise movements of the hand. With a shovel, he needs a grasp that provides more power for scooping. He will learn to change this grasp only if the circumstances require it. For example, if the sand is heavier in the sandbox when it's

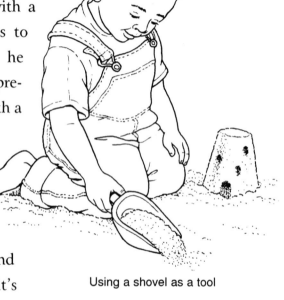

Using a shovel as a tool

wet, then he may use both hands with the shovel when scooping. The child becomes more proficient with using tools as he is able to move or adjust objects in his hands. For example, the child will learn to turn a pencil in his hand to use the end with the eraser without first laying the pencil down.

When he uses a tool, the child must be able to coordinate his arm and hand movements with his vision. His ability to plan and adjust movements of his hand in response to feedback from his eyes is necessary to repeat hand movements such as scooping with a spoon. If the food is peas, the child must see where to scoop with the spoon because the food may have rolled to another part of the plate. Vision also gives information about the size, shape and texture of the food, so an older child might chose to use a fork with pieces of hot dog. When young children begin to use scissors, they must not only be able to imitate how to hold the tool but how to use it. Cutting a circle takes very exact movements of the arm and hand guided by information from the eyes.

The child must be able to coordinate both hands together. One hand may hold or adjust the object while the hand with the tool performs the activity. When first learning to color, the child may hold the paper still against the surface of the table so it won't move. However, as his skills improve, he may begin adjusting the paper with the assisting hand. Much later, a child learns to coordinate his hands while using two tools, such as holding meat with a fork while cutting with a knife.

So a child's interest in tools is only the beginning of the journey toward learning how to use them. As you can see, there is much that needs to happen between playing with a toy hammer and actually hammering a nail into a wall. However, a little practice really will make perfect, so though you may not want to give him a hammer or pen, showing your child how to use a broom might have its advantages.

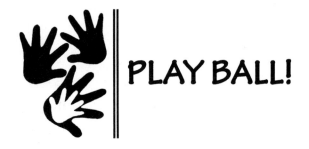

PLAY BALL!

Have you ever worked with a child who is just learning to catch a beach ball? If so, you know how much it entails. "Okay, turn toward me . . . you gotta keep your body still . . . now watch the ball . . . put your hands out . . . here comes the ball, 1-2-3-go!" Learning to throw and catch a ball is important not only because it allows the child to practice so many different skills, but because it is fun for children of all ages!

Catching and throwing a ball require many different skills involving the trunk, eyes, arms and hands. The child needs to learn

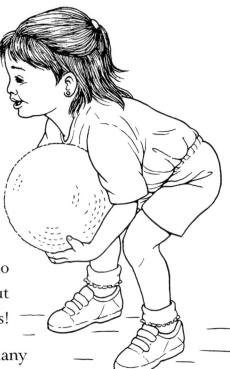

Ball play involves movements from the whole body.

how to keep her trunk still at times, but allow it to move at other times. Did you know that when she begins to throw the ball, the child's trunk is actually the first thing to move? This movement will then progress down her arm into a complex sequence of shoulder, elbow, wrist and hand movements. The child's trunk needs to be stable at other times to allow for one or both arms to reach away to catch the ball as it comes toward her. Also, the child needs to learn to use her eyes to perceive where the ball is going. This information is communicated to the muscles in her arms and body, allowing her to be in the right place at the right time to catch the ball. This is especially important if the ball is thrown to either side of the child. She needs to visually perceive where the ball will land and readjust her body and arm position to successfully catch the ball. The child needs to learn to curve her hand around the ball. This allows her grasp to be efficient whether catching a small tennis ball or a large beach ball. The child needs to learn how to let go of the ball, too. When she returns the ball to her partner, a timely release is needed so that the ball stays on target. If the release is too early or too late, the ball will not successfully reach her partner.

A child is able to throw a ball before she can catch one. Early on, throwing a ball is considered successful even if it never reaches the target. Throwing also requires the use of one arm. By the age of 1½, a child is able to fling overhand or throw a ball in a forward direction without falling down. It is not until her second year that the child is able to throw with better purpose and accuracy. You can see this when your 2-year-old can successfully throw a beanbag into a nearby bucket. In her third year, the child is able to gain even more control of where the ball will go. At this time, she can probably throw a ball straight to a friend who is 5 to 7 feet away.

Catching involves more mature skills such as using both arms together. It also requires the eyes to accurately time when the hands reach to connect with the ball. A child can catch a large beach ball with both hands from a few feet away at around 2 years of age. At around 3 years, the child is better able to coordinate what she sees with the movement of her arms and hands and can probably catch a kickball from 5 feet away. Eventually, in the child's fifth year, she will be able to catch smaller balls, such as a tennis ball, from a distance of 5 feet.

Before you begin the process of teaching your child to play catch, there are a number of things to consider. Keep in mind that different balls have different attributes and some take more skill to catch. A good rule of thumb for picking an appropriate ball for your child is to start with a larger and lighter ball, such as a beach ball. This allows more time for your child to use both her body and arms to respond to information received from her eyes. There is also more surface area to connect with on a larger ball, making it a larger target for your child's hands. As your child becomes more successful in catching, she will begin to handle smaller and heavier balls that require faster movements.

There are a number of ways to prepare your child for ball play without even using balls. Start by having your child practice clapping bubbles with both hands. This allows her to successfully learn the movements needed in catching with less emphasis on timing because of the weightlessness of bubbles. Another way to challenge your child's ability to use her eyes and hands together is to play with a lightweight scarf. Your child must continually watch the scarf as it drifts and turns in the air, and then move her body and hands to catch it.

Most of the sports we choose to play involve using our bodies to help move a ball. So whether your child becomes interested in playing tennis, volleyball, basketball or golf as she gets older, it will benefit her to practice the basic skills of controlling a ball. You don't even have to tell her that while she is playing ball she is practicing many important hand and eye skills that will prepare her for better performance on school work and in tasks around the home. Let's play ball!

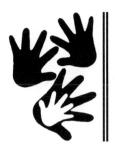

COLOR BETWEEN THE LINES

A child has to experiment with his voice before he can talk. Babbling and cooing help a baby practice movements in his mouth that later will be used to form words. A young child's hand movements when he scribbles can be compared to a baby's babbling. In fact, those scribbles have even been called "motor babbling." Just as a child's babbling turns to words, a child's scribbles turn to pictures and letters. Of course, this whole process takes a few years to complete.

A child first scribbles when he is about 1½ years old. These first marks are usually angular zigzag lines. As the child's movements smooth, these lines become more rounded marks. The child begins to draw straight lines, both up-and-down and side-to-side, when he is about 1½ to 2 years of age. Up-and-down lines usually appear first and lines drawn side-to-side appear a few months later. After the child has learned to make straight lines, he will make a circular shape. A child will typically develop a complete circle, with the end points of the lines almost touching or overlapping, just before he turns 3.

Creating artwork—whether it is scribbles, a drawing, his name or a masterpiece—depends on a number of basic skills. The child's trunk must be stable so he can control the movements of his arm and hand. These controlled movements allow the child to move the crayon in many directions. The child also must be able to coordinate the movements of his arm and hand so that he can hold the crayon and move his arm smoothly when coloring. At the same time, he must coordinate these arm and hand movements with images he receives through his eyes. It takes a lot of coordination for the child to be able to create a shape or a picture like a smiley face.

As your child begins to have more control of the crayon, you will notice the movement in his arm will progress from the shoulder to the wrist and eventually to using mostly the fingers. Initially, when your child is using his shoulders and trunk to move the crayon for scribbling, he will not rest any part of his arm on the table—just the tip of the crayon. Later, as he starts to imitate simple lines, he will begin to rest his forearm on the table surface with movement coming from his elbow or wrist. Eventually, he will be able to rest his wrist on the table and move the crayon or pencil with his fingers only. By the time your child begins to copy letters, he is likely to have already developed a mature pencil grasp using the thumb, index and middle fingers. This hand position allows him to make complex shapes and designs without having to move his wrist or arm at all. Soon the child will be able to write in small spaces, creating the turns, twists and loops that are needed in printing and cursive writing on lined paper.

Many parents wonder whether the marks on the paper have meaning to their child. The child's first scribbles are not thought to represent anything at all. However, as your child begins to draw straight lines, he is often attempting to imitate a design. As he continues to practice lines and shapes, he may start to assign meaning to the drawing after it's finished. Early on, the child's drawing will not look like what he says it is. At this point, you or other adults learn to ask rather than guess what your child has drawn.

When your child begins to create a picture that represents something he has seen, usually the picture is still a composite of the shapes he has learned, but it begins to look more like the object. A picture of a dog may be made from a circle for the head and body and sticks for the legs. We appropriately call these initial drawings "stick figures." This is an exciting milestone when your child learns to copy what he has seen. It means that his brain has become more sophisticated in coordinating his arm and hand movements with images his eyes perceive.

COLOR BETWEEN THE LINES (continued)

Many parents think that their young child should practice with pencils, crayons or markers as soon as he can hold the writing utensil. However, coloring requires many skills and the muscles in the child's hand need to be developed to a certain level before he should use standard crayons and markers. A child can develop an incorrect grasp due to early "practice" because he has been asked to use writing tools before his hand has matured. Before he is 3 years old, a child should be provided with more opportunities to

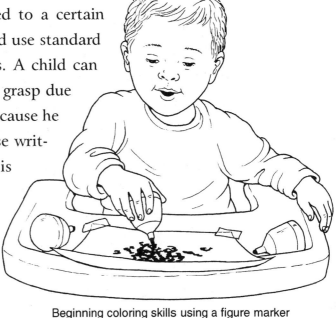

Beginning coloring skills using a figure marker

play with materials other than writing tools. Toys and objects like blocks, pegs, beads and stickers will help him strengthen his index and middle fingers and thumb without creating the opportunity for an incorrect pencil grasp to develop. If a young child continues to be interested in crayons, provide preschool crayons or shorten the stem of the crayon to 1 inch. The shorter crayon will encourage the child to use his thumb, index finger and middle finger to hold the crayon. These are the fingers used in a correct grasp.

Do you remember seeing your child's first "motor babbling?" What a thrill to realize your child is already making an impression on the world. These first scribbles are important because they lead the way for more opportunities, including scribbling on his arms and legs, the kitchen counter, the sofa, the piano bench, the bedroom wall . . .

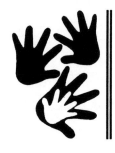

THE CUTTING EDGE

Most of us have a story about cutting our own bangs or having an older sibling cut our hair. Your own child may already have tried to cut hers. Children usually do this right before a scheduled family photo session or a special event like a recital. When a child is able to use scissors well, it almost seems inevitable that some disaster will occur.

Three years is the ideal age for most children to begin using scissors. However, even the handle holes of the smallest scissors available are too large for the hands of most 3-year-olds. When the handle holes are too large, the child tends to place most or all of her fingers into the loops of the handles. Learning wrong finger placement can lead to the habit of using a hand grasp that results in poor use of the scissors. An inefficient grasp will often cause the child to use the muscles of the forearm, which are not adept at the small movements necessary for cutting. When scissors fit the child's hand, she can properly hold them. The ideal grasp uses the thumb in the upper handle and the middle finger in the lower handle with the index finger placed outside on the bottom shaft of the scissors for stability. The ring and pinky fingers are tucked into the child's palm. A correct scissors hold uses the hand muscles that are specially designed for the small movements needed to open and close the blades of the scissors.

Cutting with scissors requires many skills that the hands of young children do not have. When cutting, the child must be able to make small finger movements of bending and extending to open and close the scissors. The child must be able to use

Using small scissors with small finger holes

the two sides of her hand separately with the thumb, index finger and middle finger being active while the ring finger and pinky are quietly tucked in the palm. The child must position her forearm correctly to align the cutting surface of the scissors with the paper. She also must be able to continually adjust the paper in the non-cutting hand.

Consider providing other activities that develop hand skills before your child is three. Many activities can address the skills used with scissors without allowing the child to develop a faulty scissors grasp. Using salad tongs or tweezers to pick up cotton balls will give your child an opportunity to practice the hand movements that are used with scissors. When you do introduce scissors, do not be in a hurry to give your child something to cut. Instead, teach your child how to simply open and close the blades of the scissors. It might be fun to pretend that the scissors are talking. Once your child is able to open and close the scissors smoothly and rhythmically, you can introduce materials to cut. At first, provide things that can be cut with one snip like straws or narrow strips of heavy paper. You then can pretend the scissors are eating. It is helpful to provide heavier paper when your child begins to be able make consecutive snips to cut 4 to 6 inches into a paper. Heavy paper provides firmness that allows the child to focus on the task of cutting rather than handling the floppy paper. Ideas for firmer materials include index cards, old playing cards, old envelopes or construction paper.

Once your child can make consecutive snips, try introducing straight lines and simple shapes. Circles are the hardest simple shapes to learn to cut. Larger shapes are easier to cut than smaller shapes. If you make the lines of the shapes thick, your child can feel more successful about cutting on the line.

When you work on cutting with your child, you might want to incorporate it into a simple arts-and-crafts project. Perhaps if you offer this artistic outlet, you can divert your child from giving someone a creative haircut.

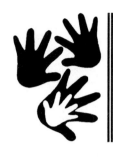

THE FINE PRINT

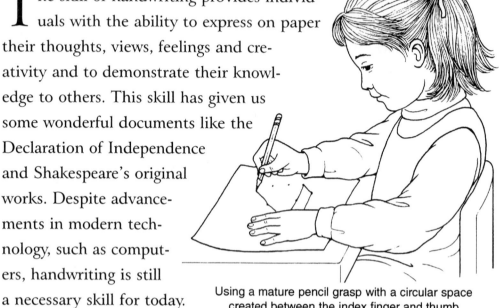

The skill of handwriting provides individuals with the ability to express on paper their thoughts, views, feelings and creativity and to demonstrate their knowledge to others. This skill has given us some wonderful documents like the Declaration of Independence and Shakespeare's original works. Despite advancements in modern technology, such as computers, handwriting is still a necessary skill for today.

Using a mature pencil grasp with a circular space created between the index finger and thumb

The ability to form letters and learn to write is one of the biggest challenges of early childhood. This stage is often when problems with hand skills become evident, if they have not been noticed before. There are so many skills that need to be in place for a child to begin to print. A child must be able to maintain stability in her trunk so that her hands are steady enough to write. At the same time, she must be able to make necessary adjustments in her posture. But this isn't all. She needs to have the same type of balance between stability and necessary movement in her shoulder, elbow and wrist. She also must be able to isolate her finger movements in her hand. Her thumb, index finger and middle finger maneuver the pencil while her ring finger and pinky stay tucked inside her palm.

There's more. Besides the stability of her posture and movements of her hands, the information and feedback from her senses must be used for coordination and accuracy of movement. Awareness of hand movement and position, obtained through touch and information from the muscles, is necessary for the child to know such things as how much pressure to apply when using the pencil. She also must know how much to move her hand to create the small marks that make up letters, and she must time those movements to form the letters fluidly. Eventually, the child will develop enough awareness to know what direction to move the pencil when she briefly looks away at the chalkboard.

Visual acuity is important for the child to see the letters, but her eyes must also be able to scan the letters in a word. Her eyes must be able to follow her own pencil when she forms the letters. The child must have the ability to interpret what she sees on a paper or chalkboard and then use a pencil to reproduce it with her hand. This is no small task. It includes the ability to understand how letters should be oriented on the paper and how the letters and words are spaced in relation to each other. The child also must be able to tell the difference between letters and numbers that look similar. Furthermore, she must plan and sequence her movements in order for her hand to form the letters. Finally, the child must be able to use her two hands together well. The preferred hand will use the pencil while the other hand holds the paper on the table and adjusts it when needed.

Prior to learning letters, a child first practices by making geometric shapes. She first may learn to make horizontal and vertical lines and circles, but by 5 years of age, she'll advance to crosses, squares and triangles.

A few children may begin to write at the age of four, but many learn at the ages of five or six. Prior to that, a lack of maturity in hand skills may lead to the child adopting an incorrect grasp and poor writing habits. Once a child is ready to write, the process can be just as confusing to the adult who is helping her as it is to the child. There are many theories about the best method for a child to learn to print. Experts debate about whether a child should learn to print using a slanted style or a vertical style. There is also disagreement about whether a beginning writer should use lined or unlined paper.

Many parents start the process by simply teaching their child to write the letters of her name. Whether you want to teach your child to write her name or teach her the rest of the letters, there are some helpful things to know. Capital letters are easier to learn than lower case letters. They are all the same height, and they all stay above the bottom writing line. They all start at the top. They also look more different from each other than lower case letters do. Compare *P* and *Q* with *p* and *q*. Capital letters are big and bold, which is a typical kindergartner's style. Letters with diagonal lines, such as *K* and *W*, are more difficult. Although they have been making horizontal and vertical lines since they were 2 years old, many children don't have the ability to imitate a simple diagonal line until the end of their fourth year. Letters that change direction mid-stroke, such as *S* and *G*, are also more difficult.

It is also helpful to consider your child's position when teaching her to print. A child-size table and a chair with a back may be better than the kitchen table. Too many distractions in the room, like the TV, will also make learning difficult. Last but not least, make it fun. Make up a song or poem about the movements needed to form each letter. If you use the same lyrics over and over for each specific letter, it will help your child remember the letter. You don't have to use paper and pencil. It might be more fun to make letters in shaving cream or finger paint. Play a game by forming the letters in the air using big arm movements. Can the other person identify the letter? The more senses involved, the better your child will learn.

THE FINE PRINT *(continued)*

Remember that learning to print is one of the biggest challenges in early childhood, so it will take time to learn it right. Remember, too, that very few important events in history ever occurred quickly.

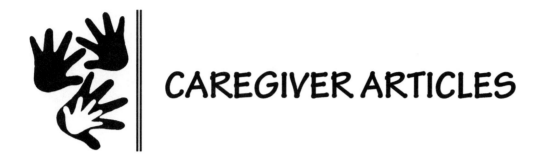

CAREGIVER ARTICLES

ADAPTATIONS FOR HAND ACTIVITIES

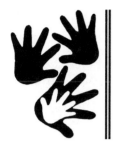

NO TIME LIKE THE PRESENT

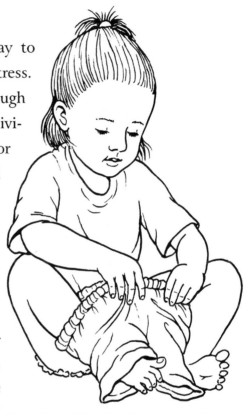

Not a lot of time in your day to practice hand skills? Don't stress. Yes, many skills are learned through structured activities, but those activities don't have to be set up or planned. At times, the best and easiest way to work on hand skills is to carefully reconsider your child's everyday activities.

Reconsider dressing. If you don't have a lot of time, pick one piece of clothing that your child can participate in removing or putting on. Pulling off clothes will use the whole hand to grasp, usually one hand at a time, while putting on

Everyday activities like dressing provide many opportunities to practice hand skills.

clothes usually means the child is using both hands together. For a higher level skill, have your child distinguish the front of the shirt from the back. This will help her to better perceive and understand information about the clothing using her eyes. When she manipulates buttons or other fasteners, your child is practicing more complex hand skills such as combining a precise grasp—using the index finger and thumb—with using both hands together.

Reconsider eating. There are many opportunities to use a variety of grasps depending on the type of food chosen. Cylindrical food such as teething biscuits or large pretzel rods require grasping with the child's whole hand. Thin foods such as graham crackers help your child use the small skilled muscles in the hand to securely hold the food as she brings it to her mouth. Placing small foods such as raisins or cereal pieces on the table or high chair tray allow your child to practice a precision grasp. This is also a good opportunity for her to work on moving objects in and out of her hand. Encourage your

Using a precise grasp to pick up a Cheerio®

child to pick up one raisin and then another in the same hand. In order to free up her index finger and thumb to pick up a second raisin, she will need to move the first raisin back into her palm, eventually releasing both raisins into her mouth. Give your child a cup or eating utensil so she can work on her grasp, using both hands together, and improving the coordination of eyes and hands. An example of this is when she stabs a piece of fruit with a fork.

Reconsider bath time. Squeezing water out of sponges or washcloths is a great way to strengthen both the powerful and the skilled muscles of the hand. Having your child grasp at toys floating by will help her fine tune the coordination of her eye and hand skills. It will also encourage her to use her whole hand to grasp with one hand or with both hands together. Pouring water from one cup to another encourages the child to turn her forearms fully. This also helps her improve her ability to move her hands in response to information from her eyes. An example is when the child learns how to position her hands to catch the most water in the lower cup. Placing shaving cream on the bathtub walls will help strengthen her arms and trunk muscles as she holds her arms away from her body to work with the shaving cream. When she draws simple shapes in the shaving cream, she is working on the isolated finger extension of her index finger as well.

These are just some of the hand skills that naturally appear in everyday activities. As you become a more trained observer of hand skills, you will discover many different ways to incorporate desired movements into your child's daily events. Remember that a child learns best when the activity has meaning for her. Learning a hand skill in the context of daily activities is always meaningful. No time to practice hand skills in your day? Don't worry. Don't sweat it. Your child can learn a lot in a typical day.

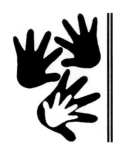

GIVING A HELPING HAND

You've probably experienced momentary frustration trying to do a task with one hand because your other hand is holding a child or loaded down with groceries. Aren't you grateful to people who open a heavy door for you or hold the receipt while you try to sign it? You know, though, that your frustration is only a taste of what your child experiences when she has limited or no functional movement in an arm and hand. So how can you help your child?

You can provide activities that encourage your child to use the movement she does have in her affected arm. But just as important, you can also make your child's daily and routine activities easier for her, much like that person who opened the door for you.

So how do you do this? Lets start by understanding how you typically use your two hands together. This may give you some insight about where your child needs help. One way you use your hands together is to hold an object with both hands mirroring each other's movement or position. This approach is called unison. An example is when you hold a large ball or box. Another way you use your hands together is when one hand holds or stabilizes an object while the other hand carries out the activity of exploring or manipulating it. This approach is called differentiated. When you open a jar, one hand unscrews the lid while the other hand holds the jar. When you write a letter, you use one hand to write while stabilizing the paper with the other. Another way you use both hands is to perform different but complementary movements at the same time. It is no surprise that this approach is called complementary. When you button a shirt, one hand pushes the button through the hole while the other hand pulls the cloth over the button. When you type, the fingers of both hands hit different keys while working together to produce words in a document.

However, if your child's affected arm provides only limited help to the more functional hand, adaptations to activities might be needed. This is where you, the parent, can help. When your child is attempting an activity where the two hands would typically work in unison, you can teach her to compensate for the other arm's limitations by trapping the object against her stomach or the other arm. Sometimes the affected arm has enough movement to pick up the object but is unable to hold onto it. In this case, you can teach your child to grab onto the affected hand with the stronger hand while wrapping both arms around the object. You may also want to look at the characteristics of the object being used in the activity. If you are playing ball with your child, try choosing a lightweight ball like a beach ball. Since her affected arm may be slower to move, adapt the activity so your child has more time to respond. Rolling or bouncing the ball may allow her to successfully use both arms. You can add handles to many objects. If you want your child to be able to pick up her puzzles, leather handles on each side of the form board may allow your child to slip the affected hand through while holding on with the other hand to carry. If your child wants to carry several small objects such as action figures, they can be placed in a container with handles or in a front fanny pack.

When your child does an activity that typically requires one hand to hold or stabilize an object while the other hand carries out the task, there are many ways she can use other body parts to assist the lead, or active, hand. She can use her legs to hold an object between her thighs. If she is trying to open a jar, she can hold the jar between her legs while her lead hand unscrews the lid. She can trap an object underneath her legs as she plays on the floor. For example, if your child is playing with a puzzle or pegboard, she can stabilize the board under her legs as she pulls the pieces out. If the child is sitting at a table, she can still use the weight of the affected arm to stabilize an object. Common household items can be used to stabilize objects, too. Rubber matting, typically used under area rugs, will keep items from slipping on a table. Clothespins, large clips or tape can tack things down. Look for toys that have suction cups on the bottom. Many children's plates have suction cups on the bottom.

Some of the most difficult activities to adapt are those that require sometimes stabilizing the object and sometimes moving the object to complete the task. When you write or cut with scissors, the assisting hand is constantly

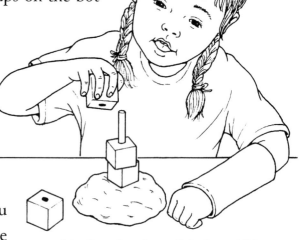

Adapting a beading activity for a child who has use of only one hand

adjusting the paper. For writing, the use of a paperweight allows more movement of the paper than taping it down does. For cutting, devices are available for purchase that can help you both stabilize and cut the paper using only one hand. When stringing beads, the assisting hand typically holds and adjusts the bead while the other hand strings. A wooden dowel in a base of play dough would eliminate the need for both hands because the beads could be "strung" on a static dowel.

When your child shows interest in an activity that uses both hands to do different but complementary movements at the same time, such as buttoning a shirt, she may need to learn a totally different way to perform the activity. There are many techniques that allow the child to be independent despite not having the use of both hands. For example, your child can learn to lay a T-shirt on her lap and pull the sleeve up first on the affected arm, then wiggle her other arm in. Once her arms

104

are in, she can pull the shirt over her head. To help her be independent, you may have to make some special purchases for your child. This may be as inexpensive as a button aid, which is a small device that will help a person button with one hand. Or it may be as expensive as a one-handed keyboard. The equipment you purchase will depend on your child's needs and your resources. You may want to seek a professional's advice before you make any major purchase.

As you can see, there are many creative and simple ways you can help your child throughout her day. Although it will take some effort, you may just find that once you start looking for ways to adapt activities, it will become easier each time. Through your effort, you are demonstrating to your child the importance of pursuing independence through creativity and hard work. And this is a lesson that will be invaluable to your child, especially during times of frustration.

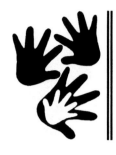

THE SETUP

Imagine sitting down to eat dinner but having your meal positioned to your right side. How would your movements be different if your meal were positioned on your left side? It might affect which hand you choose to eat with, as well as what food you choose to eat first, based on its location on the plate. Placement and setup of objects ultimately affect our movements and actions.

In much the same way, when you set up an activity for a child, you can affect that child's movements just by how you set up or place the activity in relation to the child. For example, picture your child playing with a simple wooden puzzle. If you position the puzzle on the floor rather than at the table, you are providing an opportunity for him to bear more weight on his arms. Picture it. In order for your child to reach the puzzle pieces that are an arm's length away, he must place one hand on the floor while he reaches over with the other hand to get the puzzle pieces. On the floor, the child also has the option of lying on his tummy,

This activity is set up for weightbearing on arms.

THE SETUP (continued)

propped up on his elbows. In this position, he needs to shift his weight from side-to-side in order to free either hand for reaching. Weightbearing and weight shifting make the child's arms stronger.

Similarly, just by using puzzles with small peg handles on them, you are encouraging your child to use a certain grasp. He will be more likely to use his index finger, middle finger and thumb—or the skilled side of his hand—to pick up the puzzle pieces. If, instead, your child is using his whole hand to grasp the puzzle piece, simply hold the puzzle piece in the air at his midline. The midline is an imaginary line drawn down the child's middle, from the top of his head to the bottom of his toes. When the puzzle is held in this position, he will be more likely to use the part of his hand that is closer to the midline to grasp the puzzle piece. That part of the hand is the index finger, middle finger and thumb, or the skilled side of the hand.

To reinforce use of both hands, place the puzzle pieces in a sealing sandwich bag. Your child will have to pull the bag open using his index finger, middle finger and thumb, and then hold the bag with one hand while removing the puzzle pieces with the other. If you have your child move the puzzle to and from its storage place, he will need to reach for and hold the puzzle with both hands and also hold the puzzle level while carrying it or setting it on the shelf.

Now imagine your child's favorite activity. How can you challenge him by setting up the activity differently? Being aware of not only what activities to provide, but how to present them, will help improve your child's fine motor skills.

Reproducible. © 2001 by PRO-ED, Inc.
Handprints–Pieraccini and Vance

107

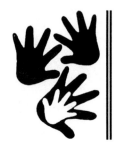

SETTING THE MOOD

Have you ever had a headache after going to a carnival or a state fair? All the loud noises of music and people, the combination of barbecue and cotton candy smells, the rides you got on with your kids and the sun beating down on you probably sent your brain into sensory overload. It was most likely fun, but you probably didn't want to do anything that required thought

Being able to change positions while playing on the floor may help a child maintain attention.

when you got home. Now remember the last time you sat through a lecture or speech where you had to fight the feeling of tiredness. The person's voice may have been monotone or soft, you may have sat in one place for over an hour and the temperature in the room may have been slightly warm. Even if it had been an interesting talk, the situation would have sent your brain into sensory shutdown. It was hard to pay attention because you just wanted to go to sleep.

In the same way that your nervous system is affected by noises, sights, smells and other sensory experiences in the environment, so your child's nervous system is affected. In fact, your child's nervous system tends to be even more reactive to what's in her environment because her nervous system is still developing. In general though, most young children are able to adapt to typical sensations around them and even thrive on them. When music is on, they will dance to it. When a fire engine with lights and a siren go past, they show excitement by pointing it out to you. As parents, we even tend to use certain kinds of sensory stimuli to affect our children's alertness and arousal states. When we want them to go to bed, we may turn off the lights, play soft music, rock them gently and cuddle them to get them to relax. However, we don't always take into consideration our children's environment when we are working with them on a new hand skill or any other skill. There are quite a few things you can do when you want to encourage your child to focus and attend to a new task. It may take some trial and error and good observation on your part to determine the optimal environment for your child.

You may find that your child benefits by decreasing visual distractions in the room, such as removing other toys from her sight and turning off the TV. You may have a room in your house that is more sparsely decorated or where toys are not typically allowed. If your child is extremely distractible, take into consideration even the colors and lighting of the room. Bright lights are associated with being awake, and we turn them down or off to relax. Soft hues of blue and green in solid colors are more soothing to our nervous systems and will help us to focus better than bold colors like red and yellow with busy patterns. However, bold and bright may be just the thing to keep your child alert. Having an area or room set aside may also help your child get into a routine of paying attention when she is there. Sometimes a small pup tent or playhouse may do—if you, the adult, can fit inside. Being in a confined area can help your child control her activity level. When you work with your child, you may also want to present only part of the activity at a time. For example, if you are working with an arts-and-crafts activity, give only the crayons first and bring out the glue later. Even with toys like blocks, it may be better to give your child only one or a few blocks at a time to stack.

Your child may benefit from controlling the noise in the area where you are working. Try to pick a time of day when it is quieter in the house, such as when other children are at school or napping. Sometimes, white noise—a fan or dishwasher—can drown out sounds such as other people talking or dogs barking outside. Music may or may not be beneficial. Rhythmical instrumental music usually works the best. If your child wants to dance to it, though, then it's probably not ideal for working on hand skills. On the other hand, songs that sound like lullabies are not ideal either because they may lull your child to sleep.

Another thing to consider is whether your child is comfortable with her surroundings. Maybe tags on her clothes or even bangs in her face are bugging her. Sitting on the floor may not provide enough support. She may be working too hard at sitting to focus on the puzzle. On the other hand, being on the floor may allow her to change positions enough to keep paying attention. Taking a snack break can also provide a change of position. Pillows or beanbags may be too soft and relaxing, or they may provide a special spot of comfort with boundaries. A booster or high chair that still fits your child may provide a comfortable seat. Other advantages of this seating are that the activity is placed on a tray where the child can see it well, and the tray provides a stable surface on which her hands can work.

So providing your child with the optimal environment may be the key to her being able to focus on learning, whether playing with puzzles or forming her first letter. It may not be easy at first to determine what type of environment your child needs. It will require you to make keen observations of her behavior. Yet, you will know that you have figured it out when you realize that both you and your child have been enjoying a certain activity for longer than you thought possible. When this happens, you are well on your way to knowing how to set the mood—despite the fact that some days you might feel that you are living in a carnival!

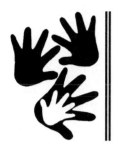

JOCKEYING FOR POSITION

Imagine the tightrope walker at the circus. When standing in such a dangerous and unstable position, she can do little more than hold onto the large white pole in her hands. When we are in an unstable position, we tend to concentrate on keeping our balance to maintain our safety. It follows, then, that when we are using complex hand skills, our bodies need to be firmly supported so that we can focus our attention on the small, specific and exact movements of the hands. Can you imagine doing such activities as threading a needle or writing with a pencil while standing on one leg?

The best supportive position can look quite different from child to child, but each will have similar components. Let's look at your child, starting from the ground up. The child's feet should always be stable, resting with the whole foot on the floor. If the child's feet are dangling in the air, the chair is too high. Simply find a shorter chair or place a large hardbound book or block of wood under the child's feet so that she can rest them comfortably.

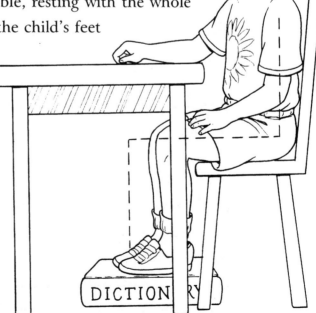

Providing seating that encourages knees level with hips and feet on a surface

111

Let's move up to the knees. When seated in a chair, the child's knees should always be level with her hips. If her knees are higher than her hips, then it would be best to find a taller chair. If the child's knees are lower than her hips, but her feet are still touching the floor, chances are the seat is too high. Again, this problem can be solved by finding a shorter chair or by placing a book under the child's feet.

Let's move up to the hips. It is important to have a stable and secure place to sit to participate in an activity such as placing coins in a bank. Make sure the child is sitting on her bottom with her hips bent and that she is not putting her weight onto her lower back. If the child often slides off the seat, a small piece of non-skid rubber mat can be placed under her bottom to provide enough friction to keep her from slipping. This non-skid material is sold at most drug and household stores as rubber place mats or as material to place under carpeting.

Let's move up to the trunk. If your child has difficulty sitting upright for long periods, the trunk should be further supported. A chair with sides or armrests might be the most beneficial tool to help stabilize the trunk. If the child is in a chair with sides and still has too much movement from side to side, simply place a rolled towel or stuffed animal between the child's trunk and the side of the chair. This will help to provide a soft yet supportive surface for the child's trunk and will encourage upright sitting. Place a small table in front of the child to create a surface on which to place an activity. This surface can also allow the child to lean forward onto her arms for more support. The height of the table should be approximately 2 inches above the child's bent elbow, or a height where the child can comfortably rest her elbows and forearms on the table without having to bend her body forward. If your child tends to lean too far forward when sitting, a table easel or standing easel can be used to encourage more upright sitting. If you place a puzzle on the easel, the child has to maintain an upright trunk to both see and interact with the puzzle.

JOCKEYING FOR POSITION (continued)

Before planning an activity for your child, it is a wise idea to spend some time looking at how your child can best be supported, so that she can do his best. Save those unstable positions for your child's big motor movements such as playing a game of kickball or hopscotch, or for the professionals under the big top!

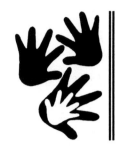

PRESENTATION IS EVERYTHING

Have you ever gone out to eat at a fancy restaurant and when the food arrived you thought, "This looks too good to eat"? If so, then you have witnessed the idea that "presentation is everything." In much the same way, we must carefully consider the best way to present an activity to a child in order for him to best learn the skill we are trying to teach.

Learning how to do a puzzle can be more important than completing a puzzle.

The most important question to ask yourself when presenting a new toy or task to your child is what do you want your child to learn with this activity. Sometimes, in an effort to help a child succeed at an activity, a parent will explain and demonstrate how to play with the toy when the child may learn better by exploring the toy and figuring it out for himself. Keep in mind that the process of learning how to do an activity can be more important for a child than completing the activity.

Depending on what you want your child to learn, you will present the activity in different ways. If you want your child to learn how to approach an unfamiliar task such as a new toy, the best way is simply

PRESENTATION IS EVERYTHING (continued)

to hand it to him, wait and watch. Let your child develop his own idea about how to play with the toy and plan the movement of his hands accordingly. For an arts-and-crafts project, simply show the child the end product and then give him the materials. Your child will need to think through the process and sequence the steps needed to complete the task. This ability to come up with an idea and plan out the movements is an important skill in your child's first attempts at a new task. You will see the benefits of this when your child attempts to imitate a Lincoln Log® building from the picture on the box.

If you want your child to work on remembering and following verbal directions, it is best to state your instructions as simply as possible, wait and watch. Your child will need to be able to listen, make sense of and recall the steps in the activity as well as plan the movements of his hands and fingers without your showing him how. This skill is important when your child is learning to sequence actions in a self-help skill such as washing his hands after only being told the steps and not shown how.

If you want to work on your child's being able to copy or imitate your movements, then simply demonstrate your actions, wait and watch. This involves your child's watching and then planning how to move to best imitate your actions. This skill is very important when your child is learning how to copy simple lines, shapes or letters from the teacher's drawing on the chalkboard.

There's another factor you should consider when setting up your child for a learning situation: how to react to your child's attempts. It is often very hard to watch your child struggle with a task. Being a loving and caring parent, you want your child to succeed in all he does. But both you and your child learn when he does not succeed right away. The child learns how to solve problems and try different approaches in order to succeed. You, on the other hand, can learn how your child takes in information and how he best learns. Is he easily frustrated? Does he ask for help quickly or does he try to figure it out? Which steps seem to be the hardest for him? The answers to these questions are helpful insights into how your child will learn new concepts in the future, and they give you information on how you can best support your child.

The best rule of thumb in knowing when to respond is to wait 10 seconds following any instruction or presentation. Ten seconds seems short, but it can be an eternity when your child is struggling. After you have counted to 10 (saying one thousand between each number!), you might simply ask your child if he needs help. If so, you can present the activity again, either in the same or in a slightly different way. This often depends on your child's current level of frustration. Sometimes just hearing or seeing the activity demonstrated again makes it click for the child. At other times, the child might need slightly more information. Often it is helpful to use words to describe what your hands look like when you are performing the activity. For example, "My fingers and thumb turn the cap, stop, move and then turn the cap again," when you demonstrate how to remove a twist cap from a bottle of juice.

When you provide instructions to your child, remember to be simple and sparse with your words. Excessive words are confusing, so get to the heart of what you mean to say—quickly! Also, keep in mind that praise is appropriate at certain times, but it can be distracting if it's given every step of the way. You do not want your child to depend on your praise or you will limit his ability to be independent.

So it is important to consider not only what activity to present but how to present the activity to your child in order for him to best learn a new skill. Whether you are preparing a meal for a small dinner party or setting up your child for learning, carefully considering how to best present the first course—or first step—will be time well spent.

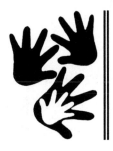

CHALLENGE OF A LIFETIME

When was the last time you worked a crossword puzzle? Have you noticed that, if a puzzle is too hard, you don't finish it because it's too frustrating or you recruit other people to help you? If it's too easy, you may become quickly bored and decide not to finish it. However, if the puzzle stretches you just a little further then your abilities, you will probably be motivated by the challenge to finish it.

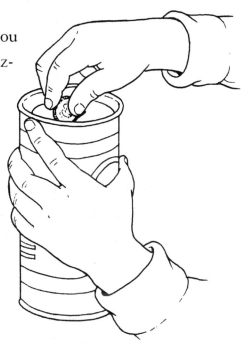

Determining your child's strengths and weaknesses can ensure the just right challenge.

When working with a child on his hand skills, it's important to keep him motivated by finding the activity that challenges just enough. At one time or another, most parents have seen the pride in their child's face after he has mastered a difficult task. It's an expression of excitement with a smile. He will look to you to see if you have observed his accomplishment. So how do you determine what will challenge your child but still provide for success? This can be harder than it seems.

You may want to start by observing your child while asking yourself a few questions. The answers should lead you to identify the just-right challenge for your child. First, you may want to ask, "What are my child's strengths and needs?" Children develop in such different ways; it's not always wise to compare your child with another. Sometimes, a professional—perhaps a pediatrician or occupational therapist—has already helped you with this question. Even so, you may want to just look at what your child currently can do with his hands, because this is the point from which you will work. You may conclude, for example, that your child shows a wonderful imagination when playing, but he has difficulty manipulating small toys like buttons or coins. He does better with medium-sized objects like blocks and pegs. You may notice, though, that he still tends to avoid activities that require him to manipulate any small toy.

The next question to ask yourself is, "How can my child be motivated to try the activities that are difficult for him?" To start to answer this question, you may want to look at the characteristics of the toy or activities that are difficult for him. Many activities can be made easier or harder by changing the toys used. Size and shape of objects are two easy places to start. For example, if your child manipulates blocks more easily than he does buttons, it may be because 3-dimensional objects are easier for him to grasp than small, flat objects. By looking through your button collection to find the thicker and bigger ones, you might find some buttons that are easier to manipulate. Then look at what part of the activity is difficult for him. Maybe he has trouble picking the buttons up from the surface of a table. If so, consider handing him the buttons one by one rather then laying a bunch on a table.

Another approach is to combine the difficult task with your child's favorite activity. An enjoyable activity can distract him from the difficult task, which may take the attention off of whether or not he can do it. You might also tap your child's inner drive for a favorite activity so he will try the difficult task. If your child, for example, enjoys imaginary play, he may be willing to play with coins while pretending to be a cashier at a store. Your child may find that what he perceived as a difficult activity is easier than he thought.

Last, but not least, provide a safe environment for trying, whether or not the results are successful. Praise your child for trying, but remember that praise can be distracting if it's given every step of the way. Never get into a power struggle if your child refuses to participate. Being matter-of-fact is often a good approach, even with praise. Sometimes just stopping the activity and returning to it later can be the best choice.

Remember the satisfaction you felt when you completed a task that challenged you, whether it was a crossword puzzle or something else? Your child needs to experience that feeling of satisfaction, too. It is difficult to see your child struggle with an activity, so you may be tempted to intervene and do it for him, or you may tend to avoid doing difficult activities with your child. Yet, finding the just-right challenge for your child is the alternative that can lead to furthering his skills and confidence, not to mention your own.

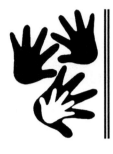

ALL TOYS GREAT AND SMALL

Next time you go to the fresh produce section of your grocery store, observe your hands as you pick and sort through the fruit. When you pick up an apple or pear, you tend to use your whole hand to grasp. When you sort through the kiwis, your hand is positioned so that you can carefully inspect the kiwi by grasping with your thumb and index and middle fingers. When picking out a cherry, you will most likely use the tips of the index finger and thumb to grasp the stem or the small, round body. Not only does size of an object affect how we use our hands, but other properties such as weight and firmness can also affect our movement. For instance, when picking up a watermelon, because of its sheer weight, you need two hands, a stable body, good shoulder strength and a strong grip. When picking up squishy fruit such as grapes, you may reach for the firm stem so you don't have to be so careful handling the fruit. You know from experience that when you hold the bunch, you can't squeeze too firmly or too lightly because the grapes may burst or be dropped. Knowing that size, weight and firmness of an object can affect your hands, what should you think about when planning activities or purchasing toys for your child? Put the toy in your hands and do a little checklist.

Check out the size. Consider the difference between your hand and your child's hands when trying out toys. What you might consider small, medium and large toys, your child might feel are large, extra large and double extra large, because of the differences in hand size. It is important to keep in mind that bigger is not always better. In fact, big objects, such as large building blocks or large puzzle pieces, can actually be harder for the young child to control because he needs to use more fingers to turn or move them. Tiny objects, such as small beads, are also more difficult because they require such precise movement of the child's fingers and thumb. In fact, the easiest-sized objects for the child to manipulate are small and are neither too tiny nor too big. We find the same thing when looking at tool use. Small scissors with small finger holes are easier for a child to manage than those with large holes, which cause the child to "fill" up the holes

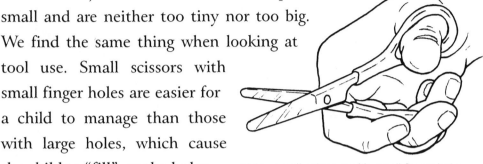

Using small scissors with small finger holes

with his other fingers. This means the opening and closing motion of the scissors will use the child's whole hand instead of the more skilled and precise movements of just the index, middle fingers and thumb. As your child learns how to manipulate tools and toys, it is most beneficial to provide him with small scissors, ¾-inch to 1-inch wooden blocks or beads, or pegs that fit nicely into his palm. Keep in mind if you are concerned about your child placing these objects in his mouth, you should consider larger objects that are 1¾ inches in size or objects that cannot fit through a toilet paper roll.

Check out the weight. Since the small child can only manage very light weight, larger solid wooden toys may be more cumbersome for him to manipulate. However, as he grows older, he will enjoy the challenge of moving heavier objects, such as putting away the canned food or pushing a stool across the floor. Light toys such as plastic blocks are easier to lift, but they don't always provide your child's muscles with enough information about weight and balance. This feedback is necessary when your child is creating a block tower or design. Keeping this in mind, toys with a variety of weights will help your child learn how to handle different objects differently. As your child's hand skills improve, he will be able to manipulate heavy and light objects with different forces from his hands and arms without a second thought.

ALL TOYS GREAT AND SMALL (continued)

Check out the flexibility. The baby interacts nicely with softer, more flexible toys such as cloth books, blocks or rag dolls because he has not yet learned how to grasp different objects in different ways. When he grasps a softer toy, the material gives, which allows him to successfully hold onto it. At this time, he can grasp a hard toy, such as a rattle, but the grasp is often tenuous, depending on where in the hand the rattle was placed. As the child grows older, his hand learns to grasp each object in a way that works best for that object. For example, the child's hands will curve slightly when holding a banana but will grip tightly around a cracker. As your child learns new hand skills, he will be more successful with firmer toys. For

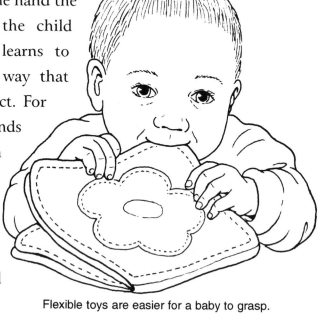

Flexible toys are easier for a baby to grasp.

example, when the child becomes interested in turning the pages of a book, he will be more successful initially with cardboard pages than with paper pages. This can also be seen when he learns to place beads on a string. The child will initially be more successful using a stiff pipe cleaner to push through the hole versus a floppy string that requires more accurate hand placement and movement. The child who is just learning to cut will be more successful cutting firmer material such as straws as opposed to construction paper. As the child becomes more proficient at cutting, he will find more flexible materials, such as copy paper, more interesting and challenging.

So next time you evaluate a toy for your child, remember your grocery store experience of how different properties of objects can cause

122

ALL TOYS GREAT AND SMALL (continued)

you to use your hands in different ways. Look at the toy from a child's perspective, put the toy in your hands and check out its size, weight and flexibility. Thinking about how your child might approach a toy or activity can help him have a successful and productive learning experience.

Handprints–Pieraccini and Vance

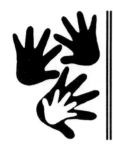

WRITING ON THE WALL

Before you read any further, understand that this is not an attempt to advocate graffiti writing or even crayon scribbling on your newly painted kitchen wall. But we do want to stress the importance of practicing hand activities on vertical surfaces for children. A vertical surface is any up-and-down plane. This could be an easel, a chalkboard, a wall, a mirror or a refrigerator door.

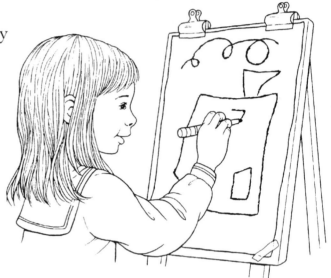

Using a vertical surface can enhance the development of fine motor skills.

Many experts believe that vertical surfaces have such a positive effect on fine motor—movements of the small muscles of the hand—development that they suggest all developing preschoolers spend at least 20 minutes a day at an easel. A mediocre activity can be made into a powerful instrument to develop these fine motor skills by simply changing that activity from a horizontal to a vertical surface.

There are several advantages to working on a vertical surface. It strengthens arm and shoulder muscles because your child's arm must move against the pull of gravity in this position. Also, she will tend to sit more upright as she writes on a chalkboard or places magnets on a refrigerator. The child's hand is best positioned to develop stability of the wrist when she is playing on a vertical surface. Picture your child

124

finger painting at an easel. The position of the slanted upright easel requires that she extend or straighten her wrist. A straightened wrist encourages a balance among the small muscles inside the hand. You can see these small muscles working together when you roll a ball of play dough at your fingertips. These movements, to bend and straighten the fingers, are the precursor to the more complex hand movements later needed for writing and cutting. Working on a vertical surface also encourages the child's thumb to move out of her palm. In this position, muscles are strengthened that will help the child use her thumb with her other fingers more efficiently to unzip a backpack, turn a lock or open a snack package. Finally, working on a vertical plane can improve your child's ability to see. Have you ever noticed that when you pick up a piece of paper to read, you generally lift it off the table in an upright angle? In this upright position, the lighting is optimal for clear focusing. Working on a vertical surface will encourage better visual attention to the activity your child is engaged in.

Unfortunately, children often play on horizontal surfaces—such as a table or the floor. When a child plays on a horizontal surface, she will place her wrists in a neutral or bent position, which does not encourage skillful use of the hand muscles. In this position, she may also lean over the activity or collapse onto one arm.

Many activities that children enjoy can be performed on a vertical surface. Your child can place vinyl static-cling pieces on windows or mirrors, or move magnets on the refrigerator. She can engage in painting activities or puzzles on an easel. On the bathtub walls, she can play with shaving cream or finger paints made especially for bath time. Chalkboards and felt boards are also natural vertical surfaces. The options are limited only by your imagination. With a little practice, you will see vertical surfaces all around that you can incorporate into your child's play. And, with a little luck, your child will stay away from being creative on your kitchen walls.

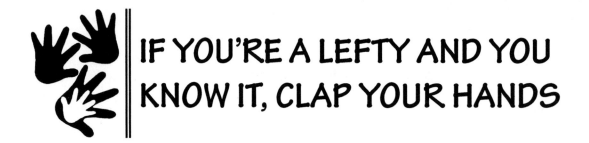

IF YOU'RE A LEFTY AND YOU KNOW IT, CLAP YOUR HANDS

Have you noticed that the world is set up for right-handed people? Most of a car's controls are on the right of the driver. In a high school classroom, all of the cutout seats have the desktops to the right for writing. However, 10 to 15 percent of the general population is left-handed. Left-handedness itself is not a disadvantage, but obviously certain challenges exist.

Handedness refers not only to which hand you use in activities that require only one hand but what role each hand takes in activities that require both hands. In two-handed activities, the preferred hand leads while the other assists. The reasons why you choose to use the left or right hand exclusively or both hands interchangeably are not always obvious.

A clear preference in handedness usually can't be observed until a child is 3 or 4 years old. However, many typical 3-year-olds still use either hand interchangeably, at times appearing to prefer one hand and then later the other.

The term hand dominance means the definitive use of one hand. This is usually not seen until a child is 4 to 6 years of age, and it appears to correlate with the development of a mature pencil grasp. If you suspect that your child prefers the left hand, realize that many people will use different hands depending on the nature of the task. You might want to observe your child in activities such as coloring, cutting or stringing that typically require the more sophisticated skills of the preferred hand.

What can you do if you are certain that your child prefers the left hand? The use of tools seems to have the most potential for frustration

Reproducible. © 2001 by PRO-ED, Inc.
Handprints–Pieraccini and Vance

for most left-handed people. The most common tools a young child uses are crayons, markers, pencils and scissors. There are several things you can do when you introduce these tools to prevent, or at least minimize, your child's frustration in school. For scissors use, it is extremely important to provide left-handed scissors. Right-handed scissors are constructed so that the bending of the fingers brings the blades together to cut the paper. What most people don't realize is that the exact same movements of the left hand cause the blades to separate. This bends the paper, causing jagged and frayed edges. The use of right-handed scissors by a left-handed child also makes it difficult for the child to see the line he is cutting, because the blade obstructs his view. You can see how the wrong pair of scissors can prevent a young child from being successful when he's learning to cut, and this can be very discouraging. As a parent, you may need to provide left-handed scissors for your child for places such as preschool, church, the community center or the baby-sitter's. You and your child might also have to continue to remind others who care for him to provide left-handed scissors when cutting is part of an activity.

If a left-handed child is taught to draw or write in the same manner as a right-handed child, he may develop a very awkward grasp. He might place his hand above the line where he is writing while bending or hooking his wrist to move the pencil. Or he might hold the pencil between all of his fingertips with the palm facing to the right while using his ring finger and pinky to move the pencil. A child often chooses one of these grasps because it allows him to see what he is writing when going from left to right across the paper. Otherwise, his hand blocks his view. This is a particular problem for the young child who needs to see what he is doing as he learns new shapes and letters. These grasps cause the child to use parts of the hand whose muscles are not designed for the small movements needed for writing. The child may experience fatigue and sometimes pain in his fingers, wrists

IF YOU'RE A LEFTY AND YOU KNOW IT, CLAP YOUR HANDS (continued)

and forearms when he relies on these grasps, particularly when writing essays as he gets older.

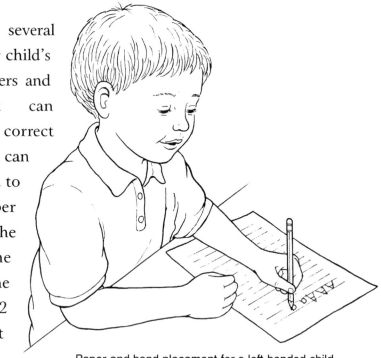

You can make several changes to your child's play with markers and crayons that can encourage a correct grasp. First, you can teach your child to turn his paper clockwise on the table, with the top middle of the paper at 2 o'clock in front of his right side.

Paper and hand placement for a left-handed child.

The paper will be parallel with his left forearm, which allows him to properly use his elbow as the pivot point for moving his hand across the paper. Also, when your child is young, you should provide him with preschool crayons. The design of the crayon encourages hand placement 1 inch above the writing tip of the crayon so your child can see his drawing. When your child graduates to standard crayons or markers, teach him to place his hand 1 to 1½ inches above the tip. You can provide cues for hand placement by providing tape or pencil grips where your child's hand should go.

Even though being left-handed can create some challenges, it does not have to be a problem if you make use of some creative and consistent adaptations. In fact, it can be a positive opportunity for you to teach your child that he is very special and unique. Learning to enjoy differences in ourselves and others is a wonderful asset.

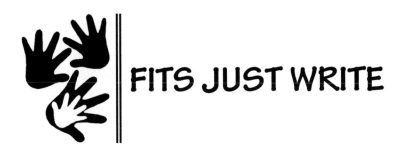

FITS JUST WRITE

You probably wouldn't dress your child in clothes that are two sizes too big for him. The holes would be too big for his arms and legs. If he's wearing pants, he might trip. If the shirt has long sleeves, the sleeves would interfere with using his hands. Shoes that are too big would make him walk with a shuffle and probably trip. His body is just not ready for that size.

However, many parents give their young children regular pencils, crayons or markers before their hands are ready for them. They don't realize that the child may develop an incorrect grasp because he has used these writing tools before his hand skills have matured. A child younger than 3 should be provided more opportunities to play with small objects other than writing tools. These can be blocks, beads, pegs or other small toys. There are many small toys that also allow a child to make fun pictures or designs without using crayons. The young child can make pictures with stickers, flannel board figures, vinyl static-cling pieces or ink stamps.

Although it is preferred that a child use a variety of small toys to develop overall hand skills, many children have a strong desire to express themselves through scribbling and drawing. Children see adults writing and drawing with tools, so naturally they want to imitate them. Writing utensils also provide an opportunity for the child to freely express himself, whether he's drawing lines and circles or a picture of the family dog. You can provide your child with writing utensils to express himself without compromising the development of a proper grasp. If you provide a shorter tool rather than standard-sized crayons, your child is more likely to use his thumb, index and middle finger, which are used in mature grasps. You need not hold back the budding artist in your young child; just provide a little guidance in the choice of artistic tools.

You can break standard crayons and chalk into 1-inch to 1½-inch pieces. Use a kitchen knife to keep the chalk from shattering as you cut it. Thicker chalk and crayons are always easier for children to hold. Sidewalk chalk, which is typically wider, can be used. You can provide your child with preschool crayons. Because these crayons are often hollow, you can put putty in the hole so your child

Using a preschool crayon

will place his fingers on the ball of the crayon, not in the hole. Children's figure markers are also a nice choice. These markers come in themes such as farm animals, zoo animals or Christmas characters. The cap is typically the creature's face. Egg-shaped chalk is a good choice, as well. This chalk is easier to find around Easter.

It may surprise you that size and shape are so important for your child's crayons, markers or chalk, but they are. Just like your child's clothes, these tools need to be appropriate for his age or stage of development. You want to promote good hand skills for later writing by providing just the right fit.

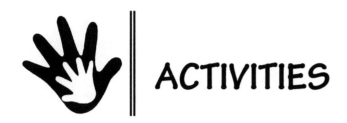

ACTIVITIES

6 MONTHS TO 1½ YEARS

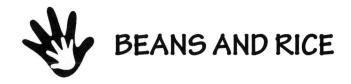

BEANS AND RICE

MATERIALS:

- mixture of dry pinto beans and rice

- small toys such as action figures (1¾ inches or greater in diameter)

- large plastic tub

- small shovels or measuring cups

HOW TO:

Preparation:

Fill the tub with 3 to 4 inches of beans and rice. Choose an area in the house with smooth flooring such as linoleum, tile or wood for easier cleanup.

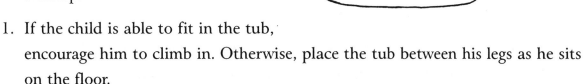

1. If the child is able to fit in the tub, encourage him to climb in. Otherwise, place the tub between his legs as he sits on the floor.

2. Show your child how to bury small toys, like action figures, in the beans and rice. Pour on additional rice and beans with the cup or shovel to cover the toy. Ask him to find the toy.

3. Now ask your child not to look by looking the other way or covering his eyes. After hiding five toys, have him find the toys.

(continued)

ADAPTATIONS:

To make this activity easier . . .

• Allow the child to watch you hide the toys.

• Allow some of the toy to stick out of the beans.

• Choose brightly colored toys that contrast with the beans so they can be easily seen.

To make this activity harder . . .

• Have the child hide toys for you to find. Encourage him to use the shovels.

• Have the child pour the beans into the cup before dumping them onto the toy.

WHY:

This activity primarily encourages . . .

Forearm pronation and supination: the ability to move the forearm back and forth between the positions of palm facing down and palm facing up. This is used when scooping food from a plate or giving a "high-5" to a friend.

Haptic sense: the ability to gather information about or identify objects through touch only. This is used when reaching in a backpack for an eraser or buttoning a shirt under your chin without looking.

Power grasp: the use of force or power on an object with the fingers and thumb acting against the palm of the hand when grasping that object. This is used when pulling a wagon with something heavy in it or opening a jelly jar.

Separation of two sides of the hand: the use of the thumb and index and middle fingers to push, poke, turn or grasp objects while the pinky side of the hand is supported in the palm of the hand. This is essential to correctly grasp a pencil or scissors.

(continued)

COMMENTS:

NOTE: An adult should supervise young children who are provided with small objects or toys. If swallowed, these objects can cause choking, which can lead to death.

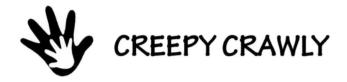

CREEPY CRAWLY

MATERIALS:

- an interesting toy

- a length of string

HOW TO:

Preparation:

Tie the toy to the string.

1. Slowly pull the toy in front of your child to get her attention.

2. Encourage her to crawl on hands and knees after the toy.

3. Allow the child to catch and play with the toy to keep her interest.

ADAPTATIONS:

To make this activity easier . . .

- Choose a toy that makes noise so your child can track the toy with both her vision and hearing.

To make this activity harder . . .

- Pull the toy under and around large, stable furniture so that the child must plan her movements to negotiate the furniture.

- Pull the toy over large, fluffy pillows that your child can crawl over.

- Encourage the child to hold a small toy in her hand that she can bang the pulled toy with.

(continued)

WHY:

This activity primarily encourages . . .

Motor planning: the ability to interact with things in the world around you in a purposeful way based on the information perceived through the senses. This means having the idea of what to with something, planning how to do it and then carrying out the plan. This can be seen when a child comes upon an unfamiliar task such as spinning a new top or playing Simon Says.

Separation of two sides of the hand: the use of the thumb and index and middle fingers to push, poke, turn or grasp objects while the pinky side of the hand is supported in the palm of the hand. This is essential for correctly grasping a pencil or scissors.

Shoulder strength and stability: the ability of the muscles in the shoulders to activate when using the arms. This is used for wheelbarrow walking, carrying heavy boxes or keeping the arms lifted to erase a chalkboard.

Trunk stability: the stability in the body's trunk to maintain an upright posture, shift weight in all directions and rotate the trunk to the left and right. This is necessary for sitting on a bench while doing a puzzle or leaning forward to pick up a toy.

COMMENTS:

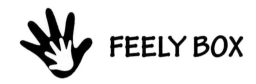 **FEELY BOX**

MATERIALS:

- shoe box

- scissors

- textured objects

HOW TO:

Preparation:

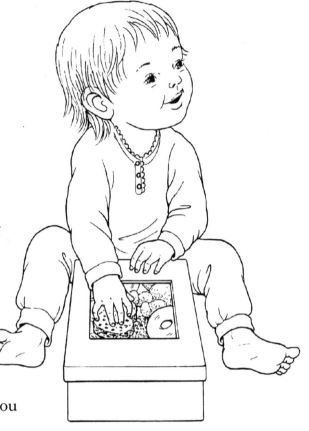

Cut a hole in the box big enough for the child's hand and objects to fit through. Find items in your house with different textures that will fit inside the box. These objects could be a furry stuffed animal, a terry cloth washcloth, a kitchen sponge, wadded paper or whatever you have in your house.

1. With the objects in the box, encourage your child to place her hand into the box to explore all the objects.

2. As your child pulls the objects out, describe the different textures using words like soft, smooth or rough. Talk about other things in the child's environment that have similar textures.

3. Encourage your child to explore the textures of the objects with her hands or have her apply the objects to other body parts like her arms and legs.

(continued)

ADAPTATIONS:

To make this activity easier . . .

- Instead of objects, apply textured material with glue to the inside of the box so that the child can feel different textures.

- Remove the lid from the shoe box so the child can see the objects she is touching.

To make this activity harder . . .

- Choose various sizes of objects so the child can identify large or small as she removes each from the box.

- Apply textured fabric to simple cardboard shapes of circles, squares and rectangles so the child can identify each shape as she removes it from the box.

- Allow the child to see the objects before putting them in the box. Then have her try to identify each object in the box before removing it.

WHY:

This activity primarily encourages . . .

Haptic sense: the ability to gather information about or identify objects only through touch. This is used when reaching into a backpack for an eraser or buttoning a shirt under your chin without looking.

In-hand manipulation: the ability of the fingers and palm to turn, twist and move an object in the hand. This is important for opening a screw top container, turning a coin between the fingertips or writing with a pencil.

Reach: the ability to extend the arm to obtain, release or hold an object. This is used when getting a toy from a shelf or catching a ball.

Release: the letting go of an object by the hand. This is used when putting dishes in the dishwasher or throwing a ball.

(continued)

COMMENTS:

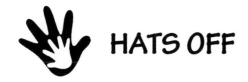

HATS OFF

MATERIALS:

- variety of hats
- full length mirror

HOW TO:

1. Place your child in a sitting position in front of a mirror and sit behind her.

2. Model putting on and taking off a hat from your own head using key words such as "hat," "on" and "off."

3. Place a hat on your child's head. Wait. Provide the key word "off" and model removing the hat from her head. Replace it on her head. After 10 seconds help your child remove the hat. Continue to place the hat on your child's head until she can remove it by herself.

4. Use this same sequence to help her learn how to place the hat on her head.

ADAPTATIONS:

To make this activity easier . . .

- Allow your child to lean against you or furnish a small seat in front of the mirror to provide supportive seating.

- Use medium-sized, firm hats like a stiff velvet hat or a straw cowboy hat.

- Have your child remove a medium-sized scarf draped over her head.

(continued)

Handprints–Pieraccini and Vance

To make this activity harder . . .

- Use tight hats, like knit snow hats.

- Practice placing and removing hats on a doll. This will require two hands to both hold the doll and move the hat.

- Using similar hats, place one of the hats on your head and ask the child to put on the hat that looks like your hat.

- Have your child remove other easy-to-remove clothing items such as sunglasses, a bracelet or large vest.

WHY:

This activity primarily encourages . . .

Forearm pronation and supination: the ability to move the forearm back and forth between the positions of palm facing down and palm facing up. This is used when scooping food from a plate or giving a "high-5" to a friend.

Release: the letting go of an object by the hand. This is used when putting dishes in the dishwasher or throwing a ball.

Shoulder strength and stability: the ability of the muscles in the shoulders to activate when using the arms. This is used for wheelbarrow walking, carrying heavy boxes or keeping the arms lifted to erase the chalkboard.

Trunk stability: the stability in the body's trunk to maintain an upright posture, shift weight in all directions and rotate the trunk to the left and right. This is necessary for sitting on a bench while doing a puzzle or leaning forward to pick up a toy.

COMMENTS:

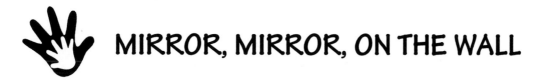 # MIRROR, MIRROR, ON THE WALL

MATERIALS:

- full length mirror

HOW TO:

1. Sit with your child in front of a mirror.

2. Make a simple hand motion like waving, clapping, patting the mirror or patting your head. Describe each motion, such as "hands up" or "hands down."

3. After each hand motion, give the child a chance to imitate you.

ADAPTATIONS:

To make this activity easier . . .

- Allow your child to lean against you or furnish a small seat in front of the mirror to provide supportive seating.

- Help your child by taking her through the motions with your hands over hers.

- Demonstrate hand motions that use only one hand, such as waving.

To make this activity harder . . .

- Pat different body parts while labeling each part.

- Play peek-a-boo by covering your eyes with your hands.

- Sing and do the hand motions to songs like "Open and Shut Them" or "Where is Thumbkin?"

- Demonstrate hand motions that use two hands at the same time, such as clapping.

(continued)

WHY:

This activity primarily encourages . . .

Eye-hand coordination: the ability of the brain to coordinate information from the eyes with the precise movements of the hand. This is necessary for catching a ball or copying a design from a chalkboard.

Motor planning: the ability to interact with things in the world around you in a purposeful way based on the information perceived through the senses. This means having the idea of what to with something, planning how to do it and then carrying out the plan. This can be seen when a child comes upon an unfamiliar task such as spinning a new top or playing Simon Says.

Shoulder strength and stability: the ability of the muscles in the shoulders to activate when using the arms. This is used for wheelbarrow walking, carrying heavy boxes or keeping your arms lifted to erase a chalkboard.

Visual Perception: the ability to perceive and understand information received from the eyes. This is used when playing follow the leader or distinguishing the difference between the letters "d" and "b" when reading.

COMMENTS:

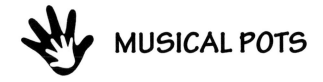

MUSICAL POTS

MATERIALS:

- pots and pans

- spoons

- music with a strong beat

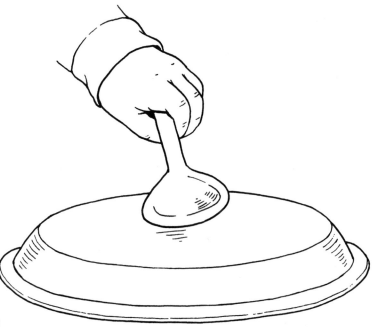

HOW TO:

Preparation:

Turn on the music or sing a song that is cheery with a good beat.

1. Have your child sit on the floor with the pots surrounding him.

2. Show him how to bang on a pot with a spoon.

3. Encourage your child to bang on a pot to the music.

ADAPTATIONS:

To make this activity easier . . .

- Have your child pat the pots with his hands instead of with a spoon.

To make this activity harder . . .

- Have your child bang smaller pots together to the music.

- Have the child bang on the pots with two spoons, alternating hands.

- Have him follow a sequence of banging on the pots, alternating one pot with another.

- Encourage your child to try to bang on the pot to the beat of the music.

WHY:

This activity primarily encourages . . .

Bilateral coordination: the ability of the hands to work together as a team. This is essential for more complex tasks such as stringing beads or tying shoes.

Eye-hand coordination: the ability of the brain to coordinate information from the eyes with the precise movements of the hand. This is necessary for catching a ball or copying a design from a chalkboard.

Power grasp: the use of force or power on an object with the fingers and thumb acting against the palm of the hand when grasping that object. This is used when pulling a wagon with something heavy in it or opening a jelly jar.

Shoulder strength and stability: the ability of the muscles in the shoulders to activate when using the arms. This is used for wheelbarrow walking, carrying heavy boxes or keeping the arms lifted to erase a chalkboard.

COMMENTS:

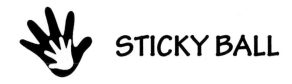

STICKY BALL

MATERIALS:

- masking tape

HOW TO:

Preparation:

Wad up a small ball of masking tape. The ball should be at least 2 inches in diameter. On the outermost layer, wrap the tape so that the sticky side is facing out.

1. Demonstrate placing the tape ball on your own hand and then pulling it off using your other hand.

2. Place the tape ball on your child's arm or hand.

3. Because the tape ball will stick to the child's arm or hand, he will reach to remove it with his other hand. As this is occurring, talk about what's happening by using words like "sticky," "hand" and "pull."

ADAPTATIONS:

To make this activity easier . . .

- Place less tape on the outermost layer of the ball to decrease the amount of force needed to pull the sticky ball off.

- Use scotch tape instead of masking tape to decrease the amount of resistance needed to pull the sticky ball off.

(continued)

To make this activity harder . . .

- Have your child follow simple directions such as, "Put the ball on your leg. Now put it on your arm."

- Put two sticky balls on the child. For example, put one on each leg. Ask the child to take the balls off using both hands at the same time.

- Place a sticky ball on a body part of your child that is out of his sight, such as on the back of his arm or on his lower back. This encourages your child to feel with his body and not rely solely on what he can see.

WHY:

This activity primarily encourages . . .

Bilateral coordination: the ability of the hands to work together as a team. This is essential for more complex tasks such as stringing beads or tying shoes.

Eye-hand coordination: the ability of the brain to coordinate information from the eyes with the precise movements of the hand. This is necessary for catching a ball or copying a design from a chalkboard.

Haptic sense: the ability to gather information about or identify objects through touch only when manipulating them with the hands. This is used when reaching in a backpack for an eraser or buttoning a shirt under your chin without looking.

Reach: the ability to extend the arm to obtain, release or hold an object. This is used when getting a toy from a shelf or catching a ball.

COMMENTS:

Reproducible. © 2001 by PRO-ED, Inc.
Handprints–Pieraccini and Vance

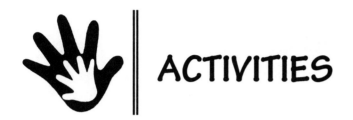

ACTIVITIES

1½ TO 3 YEARS

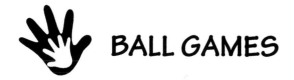 # BALL GAMES

MATERIALS:

- pair of thick socks

- laundry basket

HOW TO:

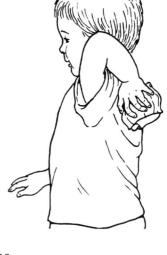

Preparation:

Lay one sock on top of the other, toes together. Roll the socks together, starting at the toe. Wrap the outside sock around the sock ball.

1. Stand about 2 to 3 feet in front of the laundry basket and demonstrate throwing the ball into the basket.

2. Have the child throw the ball into the basket from the same distance.

ADAPTATIONS:

To make this activity easier . . .

- Put a rock in the basket so it doesn't tip over if the ball hits the edge.

- Stand 1 to 2 feet from the basket.

- Stand behind the child and help him throw the ball with your hand over his.

- Put the basket against a wall so the sock ball will fall into the basket if the child overshoots.

- Put tape or lay a jump rope on the floor to help your child stay the right distance from the basket.

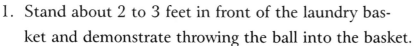
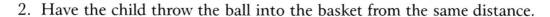

(continued)

To make this activity harder . . .

• Have the child help make the sock ball.

• Stand more than 3 feet away from the basket.

• Use a basket with a smaller opening like a wastebasket.

WHY:

This activity primarily encourages . . .

Eye-hand coordination: the ability of the brain to coordinate information from the eyes with the precise movements of the hand. This is necessary for catching a ball or copying a design from a chalkboard.

Reach: the ability to extend the arm to obtain, release or hold an object. This is used when getting a toy from a shelf or catching a ball.

Release: the letting go of an object by the hand. This is used when putting dishes in the dishwasher or throwing a ball.

Shoulder strength and stability: the ability of the muscles in the shoulders to activate when using the arms. This is used for wheelbarrow walking, carrying heavy boxes or keeping the arms lifted to erase a chalkboard.

COMMENTS:

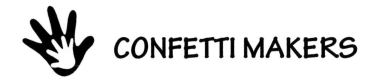

CONFETTI MAKERS

MATERIALS:

- paper in a variety of colors

- 2 pairs of scissors that have small finger and thumb holes

- self-sealing plastic bag

HOW TO:

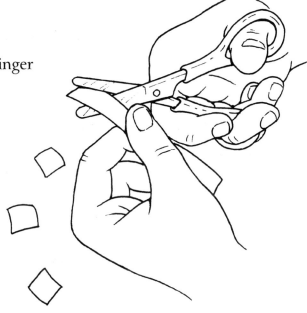

Preparation:

Cut paper into long strips approximately 6 inches by 1/2 inch. One snip of the scissors should cut the width of the strip completely.

1. Show your child how to open and close the blades of the scissors. Say, "Open" and "Close" as you demonstrate.

2. Help your child place a pair of scissors in one hand with the middle finger in the lower scissors hole and the thumb in the other. Position the child's index finger under the lower blade.

3. Demonstrate holding the paper with one hand and snipping the paper into little pieces of confetti with the other. Wait. Repeat as necessary.

4. After a small pile of confetti has been made, encourage the child to throw a handful of confetti into the air. During the cleanup phase, encourage the child to pick up each piece using the index finger and thumb. Store confetti in a plastic bag for upcoming celebrations.

(continued)

ADAPTATIONS:

To make this activity easier . . .

- Use firm paper such as old manila folders, straws, index cards or construction paper for snipping.

- Assist your child in opening the scissors blades and let him complete the snip by bringing his fingers together to close the blades.

- Hold the paper for the child.

To make this activity harder . . .

- Use thinner paper such as copy paper or tissue paper.

- Increase the width of the paper to encourage consecutive snips.

- Make dashes along the strips of paper and ask your child to "snip on the line."

- Encourage your child's ring and pinky fingers to stay nestled in his palm when cutting by placing a "cutting buddy" (cosmetic sponge or wad of paper) in his palm and asking him to hold it there.

WHY:

This activity primarily encourages . . .

Bilateral coordination: the ability of the hands to work together as a team. This is essential for more complex tasks such as stringing beads or tying shoes.

Eye-hand coordination: the ability of the brain to coordinate information from the eyes with the precise movements of the hand. This is necessary for catching a ball or copying a design from a chalkboard.

Handedness: the use of one hand more than the other in one-handed or two-handed activities. This is necessary for skilled tasks like painting a picture or cutting with scissors.

Separation of two sides of the hand: the use of the thumb and index and middle fingers to push, poke, turn or grasp objects while the pinky side of the hand is supported in the palm of the hand. This is essential to correctly grasp a pencil or scissors.

COMMENTS:

NOTE: An adult should supervise small children who are provided with sharp tools such as scissors.

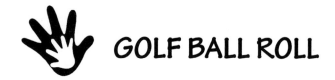

GOLF BALL ROLL

MATERIALS:

- lid of a sturdy cardboard box

- paper

- 3 colors of water-based paint

- 3 old golf balls

- 3 paper cups

- 3 old spoons or plastic spoons

- tape

HOW TO:

Preparation:

Find a cardboard box lid that your child can hold in two hands. Line the lid with paper, using tape to hold it in place. Put a small amount of each color of paint in a separate paper cup. Place a spoon in each cup.

1. Ask the child to place a golf ball in each cup of paint. Have him use the spoon to stir each golf ball until it is fully covered with paint. Encourage your child to hold the cup with one hand while stirring with the other.

2. Have the child place the paint-coated golf ball in the box lid.

3. Encourage the child to hold the box lid with two hands and practice controlling the movement of the ball.

4. Describe the movement of the ball as, "It's going to the top of your paper; now it's going to the bottom." Eventually, have the child attempt to follow instructions, such as, "Can you make the ball go side to side and stop in the middle?"

156

5. Have the child complete this activity by adding each ball, one at a time, until the child's artwork is a swirl of colors.

ADAPTATIONS:

To make this activity easier . . .

- Place one to three golf balls with paint already on them in the box on a table. Have your child use both hands to slide the box on the table top to make the balls roll.

To make this activity harder . . .

- Place stickers in different places on the paper and have your child try to roll a golf ball to the sticker, eventually learning to stop on the sticker.

- By thickening the paint with glitter or powdered tempera paint, the ball will tend to roll more slowly on the paper. Encourage your child to move the box gently so the ball will roll slowly.

- Use a smaller ball such as a marble. Its smaller surface area will be less resistant on the paper, causing the ball to move more quickly.

- Use a larger ball such as a tennis ball. Its larger surface area and increased resistance tends to slow down the ball's movement. A larger ball may also be heavier, which will require more strength to hold the box while controlling the ball.

- If the child can move the ball with good control, make shapes with the golf ball. He can make a rectangle by following the edge of the box or a circle by following the lines of a circle drawn on the paper.

WHY:

This activity primarily encourages . . .

Bilateral coordination: the ability of the hands to work together as a team. This is essential for more complex tasks such as stringing beads or tying shoes.

(continued)

Eye-hand coordination: the ability of the brain to coordinate information from the eyes with the precise movements of the hand. This is necessary for catching a ball or copying a design from a chalkboard.

Motor planning: the ability to interact with things in the world around you in a purposeful way based on the information perceived through the senses. This means having the idea of what to with something, planning how to do it and then carrying out the plan. This can be seen when a child comes upon an unfamiliar task such as spinning a new top or playing Simon Says.

Shoulder strength and stability: the ability of the muscles in the shoulders to activate when using the arms. This is used for wheelbarrow walking, carrying heavy boxes or keeping your arms lifted to erase a chalkboard.

COMMENTS:

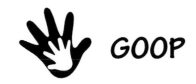 **GOOP**

MATERIALS:

- 16 oz. box of cornstarch
- food coloring
- large, square plastic storage container or dishpan
- 1 ½ cups of water

HOW TO:

1. After opening the box of cornstarch, have your child pour it into the plastic container. Encourage her to touch the cornstarch. Provide words like "soft" and "silky" to help describe the sensation.

2. Give your child 1 ½ cups of water and ask her to pour it on the cornstarch and mix it together with his hands. (*Note:* for the best consistency of goop, the mixture should be completely wet, yet thick enough to provide some resistance when grasping. You might need to add a small amount of water to get it to this consistency.)

3. Place two to three drops of the desired food coloring into the mixture. Encourage your child to mix the goop again. Continue this process until the desired color is reached and the color is blended.

4. Encourage your child to play in the goop and imitate simple movements, such as grasping the goop in one hand and releasing it onto the other, or making it "rain" down into the container.

(continued)

ADAPTATIONS:

To make this activity easier . . .

- Add more water and less cornstarch to the mixture, making the goop thinner and easier to grasp.

- Add less water and more cornstarch, and play with the mixture directly on the table surface, molding the thickened goop into a ball shape.

- Place small action figures into the mixture for the child to retrieve.

To make this activity harder . . .

- Use cups and utensils for stirring and pouring the goop.

- Add less water and more cornstarch to the mixture, increasing the strength needed to grasp and pull the goop from the container.

- Encourage your child to imitate simple letters and shapes in the mixture by using her index finger as a pencil and pushing through the goop to the bottom of the container.

- Have your child put her thumbs behind the edge of the container and, with her fingers in the goop, act like a steam shovel and scrape the goop toward the edge of the container closest to her.

- Have your child assist more in the setup process by opening the box of cornstarch or twisting off the top of the squeeze dye container and squeezing the drops into the mixture.

WHY:

This activity primarily encourages . . .

Forearm pronation and supination: the ability to move the forearm back and forth between the positions of palm facing down and palm facing up. This is used when scooping food from a plate or giving a "high-5" to a friend.

Haptic sense: the ability to gather information about or identify objects only through touch. This is used when reaching in a backpack for an eraser or buttoning a shirt under your chin without looking.

160

Isolated finger movements: the ability to move the fingers independently, whether being used individually or in combination with each other. This is necessary to rotate the dial on a pop-up toy or snap fingers to music.

Shoulder strength and stability: the ability of the muscles in the shoulders to activate when using the arms. This is used for wheelbarrow walking, carrying heavy boxes or keeping the arms lifted to erase a chalkboard.

COMMENTS:

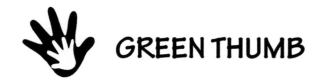 **GREEN THUMB**

MATERIALS:

- large plastic cup

- handful of small stones

- dirt

- seeds (marigold or bean seeds grow easily)

- small hand shovel

- small cup of water

HOW TO:

1. Have your child place a layer of stones in the bottom of the cup. Encourage her to pick up the stones using her thumb and index finger.

2. Help your child use the shovel to scoop dirt into the cup, filling it to 1 inch from the top.

3. Have the child poke a hole into the dirt in the center of the cup with her index finger.

4. Have her put one or two seeds into the hole, using her thumb and index finger.

5. Help the child scoop more dirt into the cup, filling it to ½ inch from the top. Show her how to pat the dirt to pack it.

6. Help your child pour enough water to moisten the soil. Set the plant in a window. Continue to water the seed and watch the plant grow.

(continued)

ADAPTATIONS:

To make this activity easier . . .

• Have your child put the dirt into the cup with her hands rather than using a shovel.

• Plant large seeds, the size of pumpkin seeds, in the dirt.

To make this activity harder . . .

• Have the child dig a small hole in the dirt with the shovel. Then have her place a small plant, root side down, in the dirt.

• Put very small seeds, the size of marigold seeds, into the hole.

• Have the child use a sprinkling can to water the seeds.

• Have the child hold a couple of seeds in her hand and, from that hand, release only one seed in the dirt at a time.

WHY:

This activity primarily encourages . . .

Forearm pronation and supination: the ability to move the forearm back and forth between the positions of palm facing down and palm facing up. This is used when scooping food from a plate or giving a "high-5" to a friend.

Isolated finger movements: the ability to move the fingers independently of each other, whether being used individually or in combination with each other. This is necessary to rotate the dial on a pop-up toy or snap fingers to music.

Power grasp: the use of force or power on an object with the fingers and thumb acting against the palm of the hand when grasping that object. This is used when pulling a wagon with something heavy in it or opening a jelly jar.

Precision grasp: the ability to use the pads of your thumb, index finger and, sometimes, middle finger to pick up or manipulate an object, with slight bending of the fingers. This is essential for picking up a raisin or unzipping a small zipper.

(continued)

COMMENTS:

PAINT YOUR WORLD WITH WATER

MATERIALS:

- paintbrushes of various sizes

- bucket

- water

- tree or concrete wall surface

HOW TO:

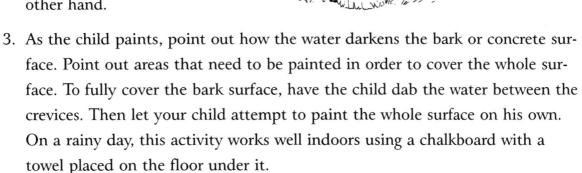

1. Help the child fill a bucket with a small amount of water. Have him carry the bucket to the surface to be painted by placing both hands around the handle.

2. Demonstrate painting on the tree or wall surface with the paint-brush in one hand while hold-ing onto the bucket with the other hand.

3. As the child paints, point out how the water darkens the bark or concrete sur-face. Point out areas that need to be painted in order to cover the whole sur-face. To fully cover the bark surface, have the child dab the water between the crevices. Then let your child attempt to paint the whole surface on his own. On a rainy day, this activity works well indoors using a chalkboard with a towel placed on the floor under it.

4. When this activity is completed, have the child carry the bucket to plants that might benefit from the remaining water.

(continued)

ADAPTATIONS:

To make this activity easier . . .

• Substitute a sponge for the paintbrush for an easier grip.

• Put food coloring into the water so the child can see his designs better.

To make this activity harder . . .

• Have your child paint lines, shapes, letters and numbers on a flat surface such as a wall. A concrete block wall with grid-like grooves is a good surface for learning to draw vertical and horizontal lines. The child can make shapes such as a cross or a rectangle by following the grooves.

• Give the child two paintbrushes—one for each hand. First, have him use both hands to paint in the same direction, either up or down. Then try more difficult moves such as having one paintbrush go up and one go down, or paint circles in opposite directions.

• Substitute a small squirt bottle for the paintbrush to encourage your child to use the two sides of his hand separately. Instruct your child to use the index and middle fingers to push on the pump while the child's ring and pinky finger wrap around the bottle to hold it.

WHY:

This activity primarily encourages . . .

Bilateral coordination: the ability of the hands to work together as a team. This is essential for more complex tasks such as stringing beads or tying shoes.

Eye-hand coordination: the ability of the brain to coordinate information from the eyes with the precise movements of the hand. This is necessary for catching a ball or copying a design from a chalkboard.

Reach: the ability to extend the arm to obtain, release or hold an object. This is used when getting a toy from a shelf or catching a ball.

(continued)

Shoulder strength and stability: the ability of the muscles in the shoulders to activate when using the arms. This is used for wheelbarrow walking, carrying heavy boxes or keeping the arms lifted to erase a chalkboard.

COMMENTS:

NOTE: An adult should supervise small children when working with water. Children can choke and even drown in small amounts of water.

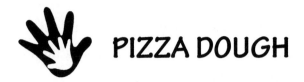 **PIZZA DOUGH**

MATERIALS:

- play dough (recipe below)

- rolling pin

- plastic knife

HOW TO:

Preparation:

Prepare play dough according to the recipe below, or use commercial Play Doh® from a toy store.

Play Dough Recipe:

1 cup salt
2 cups flour
6 teaspoons alum
2 tablespoons oil
1 cup hot water
4 packages dry Kool-Aid®
Mix dry ingredients. Add oil and hot water. Mix to a workable consistency.

1. Encourage your child to use both hands to roll a medium-sized piece of play dough into a hot-dog-like shape on the table.

2. Have your child use the rolling pin to flatten the dough on the table as if making a "pizza."

3. Using your index finger, demonstrate to your child how to poke small holes in the dough to prepare for toppings. Encourage your child to imitate your movements.

(continued)

4. Have your child pick off small pieces of play dough from the container and place them into the holes. Help him describe the pretend pizza toppings by asking questions such as, "Are you putting tomatoes on your pizza?"

5. Have your child use the plastic knife to cut slices of pizza for all who wish to be served.

ADAPTATIONS:

To make this activity easier. . .

- Have your child pat the play dough into a flat shape with his hands.

- Use items for the toppings that are firm and easier to manipulate, such as beads, dried noodles or beans.

To make this activity harder. . .

- Encourage your child to roll the play dough into a ball, creating a more circular pizza when it is flattened.

- Have your child roll the small pieces for the toppings into small balls, using the tips of his index finger, middle finger and thumb.

- Have your child assist in making the play dough.

- Have your child place beads as toppings on the pizza and then create a calzone by folding the pizza in half. Then encourage him to find the hidden toppings by digging and grasping with his index finger, middle finger and thumb.

WHY:

This activity primarily encourages . . .

Bilateral coordination: the ability of the hands to work together as a team. This is essential for more complex tasks such as stringing beads or tying shoes.

Eye-hand coordination: the ability of the brain to coordinate information from the eyes with precise movements of the hands. This is necessary for catching a ball or copying a design from a chalkboard.

(continued)

Isolated finger movements: the ability to move the fingers separately, whether being used individually or in combination with each other. This is necessary to rotate the dial of a pop-up toy or snap fingers to music.

Precision grasp: the ability to use the pads of your thumb, index finger and, sometimes, middle finger to pick up or manipulate an object, with slight bending of the fingers. This is essential for picking up a raisin or unzipping a small zipper.

COMMENTS:

NOTE: An adult should supervise young children who are provided with small objects or toys. If swallowed, these objects can cause choking, which can lead to death.

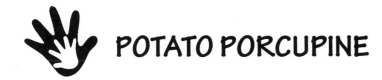

POTATO PORCUPINE

MATERIALS:

- potato
- toothpicks

HOW TO:

1. Demonstrate sticking toothpicks into the potato to make the quills of a pretend porcupine.

2. Encourage your child to hold the potato still on the table surface with one hand and push a quill into the porcupine with the other hand, using the pads of the index finger and thumb.

3. To add eyes, a nose or mouth, secure other foods to the potato with the tooth-picks.

ADAPTATIONS:

To make this activity easier . . .

- To make the potato softer, peel it or put it in the microwave for a few minutes. Be sure it is cool before giving it to the child.

- Use play dough instead of the potato for less resistance and easier penetration of the toothpick into the porcupine body.

To make this activity harder . . .

- Use a variety of vegetables or fruit for different amounts of resistance. Squash, cucumber, pear or kiwi will work. Finish the project by eating it (without the toothpicks)!

(continued)

- Help your child tuck his pinky and ring finger into his palm for stability. Place a piece of potato in the child's hand while saying, "Hold on to that!"

- Have the child use colored toothpicks or toothpicks with pompoms on them. Decorate your own potato with certain colors of toothpicks and ask your child to imitate the design.

WHY:

This activity primarily encourages . . .

Bilateral coordination: the ability of the hands to work together as a team. This is essential for more complex tasks such as stringing beads or tying shoes.

Precision grasp: the ability to use the pads of your thumb, index finger and, sometimes, middle finger to pick up or manipulate an object, with slight bending of the fingers. This is essential for picking up a raisin or unzipping a small zipper.

Separation of two sides of the hand: the use of the thumb, index finger and middle finger to push, poke, turn or grasp objects while the pinky side of the hand is supported in the palm of the hand. This is essential to correctly grasp a pencil or scissors.

Shoulder strength and stability: the ability of the muscles in the shoulders to activate when using the arms. This is used for wheelbarrow walking, carrying heavy boxes or keeping the arms lifted to erase a chalkboard.

COMMENTS:

NOTE: An adult should supervise young children who are provided with small objects or toys. If swallowed, these objects can cause choking, leading to death.

PUTTING MONEY IN THE BANK

MATERIALS:

- 15 to 20 quarters (or poker chips for a younger child)

- a plastic self-sealing sandwich bag

- container with plastic lid such as a coffee can or cylindrical raisin container (the bank)

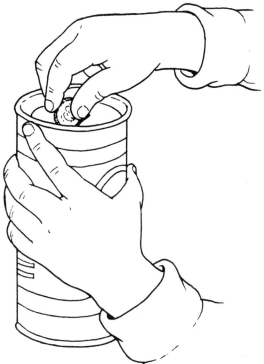

HOW TO:

Preparation:

Cut a slit in the plastic lid that is slightly longer than the diameter of a quarter. To make the container more playful, decorate it with contact paper or fun stickers. If possible, use a metal container because some children enjoy hearing the sounds of coins inside the container.

1. Give your child the sandwich bag with quarters inside. Ask her to take the money out of the bag and put it in the bank. Encourage her to use one hand to hold the bag and the other to reach inside for the coin.

2. Place the container so the slot is horizontal to the child. Encourage her to stabilize the container with one hand while placing the coin in the bank with the other.

ADAPTATIONS:

To make this activity easier . . .

- Make the slot much larger than the coin by cutting a rectangle in the lid.

- Cut a circular opening in the lid and use round objects such as pompoms or small rubber balls.

- Use larger objects such as film canisters or blocks.

To make this activity harder . . .

- Cut the slot equal to the size of the coin, requiring the child to wiggle the coin to get it through the slot, like wiggling a button through a buttonhole on a shirt.

- Place three coins on the table and ask the child to pick up the coins one at a time with one hand, keeping them in the hand. Once the coins are in the child's palm, have her put the coins in the bank using only that hand.

- Place a coin in the child's palm to be held there with the ring and pinky fingers. Tell her, "Don't drop it!" while she is placing the coins in the bank with the other fingers of the same hand.

- Once your child has mastered placing the coins in a horizontal slot, lay the container on its side so that the slot is vertical to the child. Demonstrate how to place the coin with this new orientation.

WHY:

This activity primarily encourages . . .

Eye-hand coordination: the ability of the brain to coordinate information from the eyes with the precise movements of the hand. This is necessary for catching a ball or copying a design from a chalkboard.

In-hand manipulation: the ability of the fingers and palm to turn, twist and move an object in the hand. This is important for opening a screw-top container, turning a coin between the fingertips or writing with a pencil.

Precision grasp: the ability to use the pads of your thumb, index finger and, sometimes, middle finger to pick up or manipulate an object, with slight bending of the fingers. This is essential for picking up a raisin or unzipping a small zipper.

(continued)

Separation of two sides of the hand: the use of the thumb, index finger and middle finger to push, poke, turn or grasp objects while the pinky side of the hand is supported in the palm of the hand. This is essential to correctly grasp a pencil or scissors.

COMMENTS:

NOTE: An adult should supervise young children who are provided with small objects or toys. If swallowed, these objects can cause choking, leading to death.

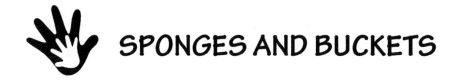 **SPONGES AND BUCKETS**

MATERIALS:

- 2 kitchen sponges

- water

- 2 small buckets or bowls

HOW TO:

1. Fill one of the buckets a third full of water. Have the child assist in carrying the bucket to an outside area.

2. Demonstrate how to place a sponge in the bucket of water and fill the sponge with water.

3. Show the child how to move the full sponge to the other bucket and then squeeze the water out of the sponge and into the bucket.

4. Encourage your child to move the water from the first to the second bucket using the sponge.

ADAPTATIONS:

To make this activity easier . . .

- Using just one bucket, encourage your child to "make rain." Show her how to fill, lift and then squeeze the sponge, releasing the water from the sponge back into the bucket.

- Cut the kitchen sponge in half, allowing the child to use just one instead of two hands.

- Give your child a small cup and have her scoop the water to move it from one bucket to the other.

(continued)

176

To make this activity harder . .

- Use a variety of different sizes and densities of sponges, such as a car sponge. The larger and denser sponges will take more pressure to squeeze than the smaller and lighter sponges.

- Substitute a washcloth for the sponge. The larger, less firm material requires better skill to manipulate with both hands.

- Instruct and encourage your child to let each hand take a turn to squeeze out the sponge by itself.

WHY:

This activity primarily encourages . . .

Bilateral coordination: the ability of the hands to work together as a team. This is essential for more complex tasks such as stringing beads or tying shoes.

Eye-hand coordination: the ability of the brain to coordinate information from the eyes with the precise movements of the hand. This is necessary for catching a ball or copying a design from a chalkboard.

Power grasp: the use of force or power on an object with the fingers and thumb acting against the palm of the hand when grasping that object. This is used when pulling a wagon with something heavy in it or opening a jelly jar.

Release: the letting go of an object by the hand. This is used when putting dishes in the dishwasher or throwing a ball.

COMMENTS:

NOTE: An adult should supervise small children when working with water. Children can choke and even drown in small amounts of water.

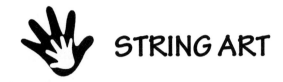

STRING ART

MATERIALS:

- paper

- newspaper

- paint smock or old shirt

- 4 colors of paint in bowls

- string of different lengths

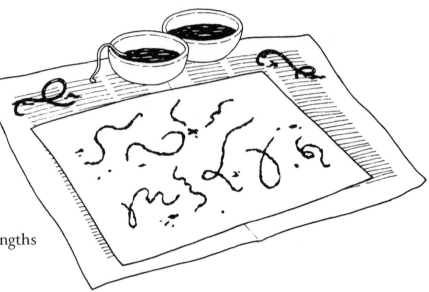

HOW TO:

Preparation:

Set out string pieces, paper and paint in bowls.

1. Encourage your child to pick up the string between the pads of his thumb and index finger.

2. Have him dip the string in a bowl of paint.

3. Instruct him to lay the string on the paper to leave the imprint of the string, and then remove it.

4. Have the child put used string on the newspaper to be thrown away.

5. Encourage your child to lay another string that has been dipped in a different color on the paper.

6. Have him continue until he has a fun design.

(continued)

ADAPTATIONS:

To make this activity easier . . .

• Instead of string, use a pipe cleaner, leather string or uncooked spaghetti in order to have more control of placement on the paper.

• Use thicker string, such as yarn, that can be more easily grasped.

• Allow the child to randomly place the string with no definite pattern.

• Use shorter pieces of string that require less controlled placement on the paper.

To make this activity harder . . .

• Encourage the child to make shapes, letters or even pictures on the paper.

• Use longer pieces of string that require more controlled placement on the paper.

• Have the child fold the paper in half, open the paper, place the string on one side, then fold the paper again to create the string design on both sides.

WHY:

This activity primarily encourages . . .

Eye-hand coordination: the ability of the brain to coordinate information from the eyes with the precise movements of the hand. This is necessary for catching a ball or copying a design from a chalkboard.

Precision grasp: the ability to use the pads of your thumb, index finger and, sometimes, middle finger to pick up or manipulate an object, with slight bending of the fingers. This is essential for picking up a raisin or unzipping a small zipper.

Reach: the ability to extend the arm to obtain, release or hold an object. This is used when getting a toy from a shelf or catching a ball.

(continued)

Separation of two sides of the hand: the use of the thumb and index and middle fingers to push, poke, turn or grasp objects while the pinky side of the hand is supported in the palm of the hand. This is essential to correctly grasp a pencil or scissors.

COMMENTS:

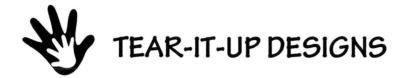 **TEAR-IT-UP DESIGNS**

MATERIALS:

- scrap construction paper or lunch bag

- glue

HOW TO:

1. Demonstrate how to rip paper. Show your child how one hand moves away from you and one hand moves toward you when ripping.

2. Have your child place his hands at the top of a medium-sized piece of paper. Place your hands over his hands and demonstrate how to rip paper. Make sure your child is using the pads of the fingers and thumbs rather than a whole-hand grasp when ripping.

3. Continue ripping smaller and smaller pieces of paper.

4. Put glue on a paper surface such as a lunch bag or construction paper. Place the small paper pieces on the larger paper to create a design or add detail to a picture.

ADAPTATIONS:

To make this activity easier . . .

- Put colored tabs of tape or dots on the paper to help the child know where to place his fingers.

- Use narrow strips of paper instead of large pieces.

To make this activity harder . . .

- Use different types of paper such as tissue paper, newspaper or magazines. Thin paper is harder to control, and thick paper provides more resistance to the fingers and thumb.

- Have the child tear out simple shapes such as circles or squares.

WHY:

This activity primarily encourages . . .

Bilateral coordination: the ability of the hands to work together as a team. This is essential for more complex tasks such as stringing beads or tying shoes.

Forearm pronation and supination: the ability to move the forearm back and forth between the positions of palm facing down and palm facing up. This is used when scooping food from a plate or giving a "high-5" to a friend.

Precision grasp: the ability to use the pads of your thumb, index finger and, sometimes, middle finger to pick up or manipulate an object, with slight bending of the fingers. This is essential for picking up a raisin or unzipping a small zipper.

Separation of two sides of the hand: the use of the thumb and index and middle fingers to push, poke, turn or grasp objects while the pinky side of the hand is supported in the palm of the hand. This is essential to correctly grasp a pencil or scissors.

COMMENTS:

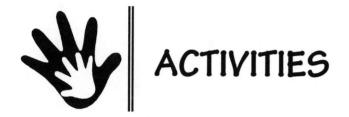

ACTIVITIES

3 TO 5 YEARS

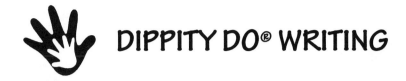 DIPPITY DO® WRITING

MATERIALS:

- tube of hair gel

- 1-gallon self-sealing plastic bag

HOW TO:

1. While you hold open the plastic bag, encourage your child to squeeze the hair gel into the bag. Seal the bag.

2. Encourage the child to squeeze, pat and press the bag.

3. Lay the gel bag on a flat surface and, using your index finger like a pencil, model simple impressions in the gel such as dots, simple lines or shapes.

4. Erase the image by gently patting on the surface. Encourage the child to imitate your impressions.

ADAPTATIONS:

To make this activity easier . . .

- Use darker colors of hair gel such as blue or green, or add food dye, and place the gel bag on top of white paper for better contrast when drawing designs.

- Draw lines and simple shapes on white paper, then place the gel bag on top of the paper. Have the child trace the shapes.

To make this activity harder . . .

- Use lighter colors of hair gel such as yellow or pink to provide less contrast. This will cause your child to rely more heavily on information about the shape from his hands rather than from his eyes.

- Have your child hold onto a pencil and press the gel bag with the eraser end.

- Have your child practice first tracing, then copying, then creating letters in the gel.

Handprints–Pieraccini and Vance

WHY:

This activity primarily encourages . . .

Eye-hand coordination: the ability of the brain to coordinate information from the eyes with the precise movements of the hand. This is necessary for catching a ball or copying a design from a chalkboard.

Haptic sense: the ability to gather information about or identify objects through touch. This is used when reaching in a backpack for an eraser or buttoning a shirt under your chin without looking.

Isolated finger movements: the ability to move the fingers independently, whether fingers are being used individually or in combination with each other. This is necessary to rotate the dial on a pop-up toy or snap fingers to music.

Visual Perception: the ability to perceive and understand information received from the eyes. This is used when playing follow-the-leader or distinguishing the difference between the letters "d" and "b" when reading.

COMMENTS:

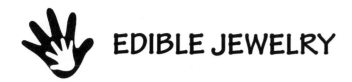

EDIBLE JEWELRY

MATERIALS:

- circular cereal (Cheerios®, Fruit Loops®)

- tape

- yarn

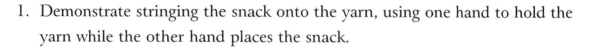

HOW TO:

Preparation:

Knot one end of the yarn and create a "needle" on the other end by tightly wrapping 1 to 1½ inches of tape around it.

1. Demonstrate stringing the snack onto the yarn, using one hand to hold the yarn while the other hand places the snack.

2. Encourage your child to use his thumb and index and middle fingers to hold the snack as he strings it onto the yarn. To begin, hand the snack to your child by holding it in the air in front of him. When he can use these fingers well, place the remaining snacks on the table. Encourage your child to also use the pads of his index finger and thumb to hold the yarn.

3. When the string is full, tie the ends together and invite the child to try on the necklace or bracelet in front of a mirror.

ADAPTATIONS:

To make this activity easier . . .

- Instead of yarn, use a pipe cleaner, a leather string or uncooked spaghetti to give the child more control when he pushes the snacks onto it.

- Instead of cereal, use larger objects such as pretzels or beads, which are easier to hold.

- Teach your child to remove the objects from the string first and then to string them back on.

To make this activity harder . . .

- Use a variety of thin or loose "strings" such as fishing line or thread with tape on the end.

- To create different challenges, use a variety of objects found around the house such as noodles, cut-up straws, buttons, tinker toys and bells. With long or narrow beads such as noodles or cut-up straws, the child must get the string into a small hole and push the yarn farther down the object.

- Place 5 to 10 different snacks on a string and ask your child to copy your jewelry design on his string. For example, a pattern could be 2 noodles, 1 yellow Fruit Loop® and 3 pretzels.

- Ask your child to remove one snack at a time from the yarn and hold it in his hand until he has at least three snacks hidden in his palm.

WHY:

This activity primarily encourages . . .

Bilateral coordination: the ability of the hands to work together as a team. This is essential for more complex tasks such as stringing beads or tying shoes.

Eye-hand coordination: the ability of the brain to coordinate information from the eyes with the precise movements of the hand. This is necessary for catching a ball or copying a design from a chalkboard.

In-hand manipulation: the ability of the fingers and palm to turn, twist and move an object in the hand. This is important for opening a screw-top container, turning a coin between the fingertips or writing with a pencil.

Precision grasp: the ability to use the pads of your thumb, index finger and, sometimes, middle finger to pick up or manipulate an object, with slight bending of the fingers. This is essential for picking up a raisin or unzipping a small zipper.

(continued)

COMMENTS:

NOTE: An adult should supervise small children when provided with small objects or toys. If swallowed, these objects can cause choking, leading to death.

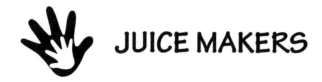 **JUICE MAKERS**

MATERIALS:

- electric citrus juicer
- 6 to 8 oranges
- knife
- adult-sized and child-sized cups

HOW TO:

Preparation:

Cut the oranges into halves.

1. Show the child how to hold the juicer's handle with one hand and the orange with the other. Holding the orange with your whole hand, press the orange onto the cone-shaped juicer.

2. Encourage the child to imitate your movements. Provide verbal instruction and physically help her as needed.

3. Pour the juice into glasses and enjoy the freshly squeezed drink!

ADAPTATIONS:

To make this activity easier . . .

- Place your hand over the child's hand to position the orange on the juicer.
- Stabilize the juicer by placing it on a non-skid mat, freeing both hands to hold the orange while juicing.

To make this activity harder . . .

- Have the child switch hands to place and press the orange.
- Have the child pour the juice into large and small cups.

- Encourage the child to squeeze the oranges first in her hands and then use the juicer to extract the remaining juice.

WHY:

This activity primarily encourages . . .

Bilateral coordination: the ability of the hands to work together as a team. This is essential for more complex tasks such as stringing beads or tying shoes.

Handedness: the use of one hand more than the other in one-handed or two-handed activities. This is necessary for skilled tasks like painting a picture or cutting with scissors.

Power grasp: the use of force or power on an object with the fingers and thumb acting against the palm of the hand when grasping that object. This is used when pulling a wagon with something heavy in it or opening a jelly jar.

Shoulder strength and stability: the ability of the muscles in the shoulders to activate when using the arms. This is used for wheelbarrow walking, carrying heavy boxes or keeping the arms lifted to erase a chalkboard.

COMMENTS:

NOTE: An adult should always supervise small children's use of an electrical appliance.

FEEDING OUR FURRY FRIENDS

MATERIALS:

- 2 stuffed animals

- 2 small margarine containers ("bowls")

- 2 handfuls of different kinds of cereal

- small tongs*

    *Tongs can be made from two tongue depressors attached to a small piece of wood. You may use tongs from your kitchen, or you can find them in a number of children's games.

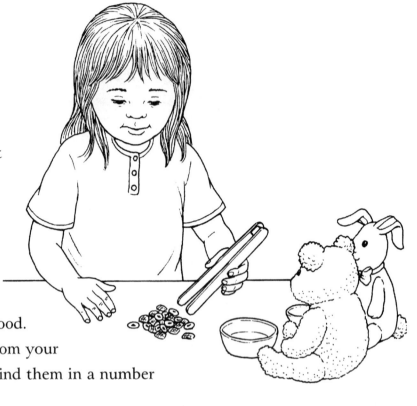

HOW TO:

Preparation:

Combine the two different kinds of cereal in a pile on the table. Instruct the child to place each stuffed animal behind a margarine container.

1. Demonstrate how to close and open the tongs using just one hand, with the tips of your fingers and thumb on the tong's surface. Have the child try opening and closing the tongs.

2. Once the child is successful with opening and closing the tongs, demonstrate picking up a piece of cereal. Have her place one type of cereal in the bowl in front of the first stuffed animal and the other type of cereal in the bowl in front of the second stuffed animal.

192

3. Encourage the child to continue feeding the animals in this way until all the food is gone.

ADAPTATIONS:

To make this activity easier . . .

- Have the child place only one type of cereal in one bowl.

- Have the child use her hands instead of the tongs to sort the food.

- Use larger foods such as small pretzels or marshmallows.

To make this activity harder . . .

- Have the child sort up to 6 different cereals in 6 different bowls.

- Use small containers, encouraging the child to have better accuracy when placing the food.

- Place a piece of cereal or a cosmetic sponge in the palm of the child's hand and ask her to hold it with the ring finger and pinky while operating the tongs with the index finger, middle finger and thumb.

- As the child gets more proficient with the tongs, have her try this activity using chopsticks that are held together with a rubber band around the top.

WHY:

This activity primarily encourages . . .

Eye-hand coordination: the ability of the brain to coordinate information from the eyes with the precise movements of the hand. This is necessary for catching a ball or copying a design from a chalkboard.

Motor planning: the ability to interact with things in the world around you in a purposeful way based on the information perceived through the senses. This means having the idea of what to with something, planning how to do it and then carrying out the plan. This can be seen when a child comes upon an unfamiliar task such as spinning a new top or playing Simon Says.

(continued)

Reach: the ability to extend the arm to obtain, release or hold an object. This is used when getting a toy from a shelf or catching a ball.

Separation of two sides of the hand: the use of the thumb and index and middle fingers to push, poke, turn or grasp objects while the pinky side of the hand is supported in the palm of the hand. This is essential to correctly grasp a pencil or scissors.

COMMENTS:

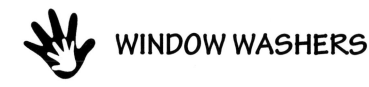

WINDOW WASHERS

MATERIALS:

- pump-type squirt bottles

- rags

- squeegee

- bucket

- water

- outside sliding glass door or window within child's reach

HOW TO:

1. Help your child fill a bucket with enough water to fill the squirt bottle. This does not have to be more than a few inches deep. Have the child carry the bucket with two hands to the window.

2. Remove the top from the bottle. Demonstrate how to submerge the squirt bottle in the water to fill it. Let her place a bottle in the bucket and hold it down to fill it. When the bottle is full, screw the top on again. Dump the remaining water out of the bucket.

3. Show your child how to spray the window with the squirt bottle. Instruct her to use her index and middle fingers to push on the pump while her ring finger and pinky wrap around the bottle to hold it.

4. Show her how to use the squeegee and rags with adequate pressure to dry the window.

(continued)

ADAPTATIONS:

To make this activity easier...

- For an easier grip, substitute a sponge for the squirt bottle.

- Use rags only to dry the window.

- Have her squirt only the bottom half of the window or a part of the window.

- Help your child carry the bucket by the handle to the window.

To make this activity harder...

- Have your child unscrew the top from the bottle before filling it with water.

- Have her move the squeegee from side to side across the window as well as up and down. You could even make simple designs like crosses and squares.

- Give the child two squirt bottles—one for each hand—so she can squirt the water simultaneously with both hands.

- Encourage her to cover a large area of the window, including some of the upper half.

WHY:

This activity primarily encourages. . .

Power grasp: the use of force or power on an object with the fingers and thumb acting against the palm of the hand when grasping that object. This is used when pulling a wagon with something heavy in it or opening a jelly jar.

Reach: the ability to extend the arm to obtain, release or hold an object. This is used when getting a toy from a shelf or catching a ball.

Separation of two sides of the hand: the use of the thumb and index and middle fingers to push, poke, turn or grasp objects while the pinky side of the hand is supported in the palm of the hand. This is essential to correctly grasp a pencil or scissors.

Shoulder strength and stability: the ability of the muscles in the shoulders to activate when using the arms. This is used for wheelbarrow walking, carrying heavy boxes or keeping the arms lifted to erase the chalkboard.

196

COMMENTS:

NOTE: An adult should supervise small children when working with water. Children can choke and even drown in small amounts of water.

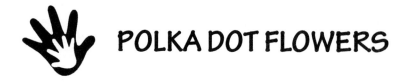 # POLKA DOT FLOWERS

MATERIALS:

- plastic eyedroppers
- colored food dye
- small containers of water
- coffee filters

HOW TO:

1. Have the child help you squeeze 1 to 3 drops of dye into the water. Use darker colors of food dye to provide a strong contrast between the dyed water and the clear plastic tubing of the eyedropper.

2. Encourage the child to practice squeezing water in and out of the eyedropper. Have her use the pads of her fingers when she pinches the eyedropper.

3. Once the child understands how to control the eyedropper, begin to dye the coffee filters with different colors to make tie-dyed flowers.

ADAPTATIONS:

To make this activity easier . . .

- Teach your child to use the eyedropper by playing with the colored water in an old ice cube container, mixing colors together. Or have her use the eyedropper to give toy figurines "showers."

- Fill the eyedropper, then hand it to the child so she can squeeze the water onto the filter.

- Use containers with large openings such as a small mixing bowl for the child to access the colored water.

(continued)

To make this activity harder . . .

- Use containers with small openings to encourage increased accuracy in placing the eyedropper into the container to retrieve the liquid.

- Ask the child to let only one drop out of the eyedropper at a time. Counting the drops out loud will give her more feedback.

- Use a variety of sizes of eyedroppers noting that each one feels different and requires slightly different pressure.

- Add a thickener such as applesauce to the colored liquid.

- Use containers of water with twist or pull lids. Encourage your child to stabilize the container with one hand and twist or pull off the lid with the other.

- When dyeing the coffee filter, give verbal cues such as, "Put a yellow dot in the middle of your flower, now on top of your flower." Point, when necessary, to help the child.

WHY:

This activity primarily encourages . . .

Handedness: the use of one hand more than the other in one-handed or two-handed activities. This is necessary for skilled tasks like painting a picture or cutting with scissors.

Precision grasp: the ability to use the pads of one's thumb, index finger and, sometimes, middle finger to pick up or manipulate an object, with slight bending of the fingers. This is essential for picking up a raisin or unzipping a small zipper.

Release: the letting go of an object by the hand. This is used when putting dishes in the dishwasher or throwing a ball.

Separation of two sides of the hand: the use of the thumb and index and middle fingers to push, poke, turn or grasp objects while the pinky side of the hand is supported in the palm of the hand. This is essential to correctly grasp a pencil or scissors.

(continued)

COMMENTS:

NOTE: An adult should supervise small children when provided with small objects or toys. If swallowed, these objects can cause choking, leading to death.

LACING THROUGH SWISS CHEESE

MATERIALS:

- laundry basket

- yarn

- tape

HOW TO:

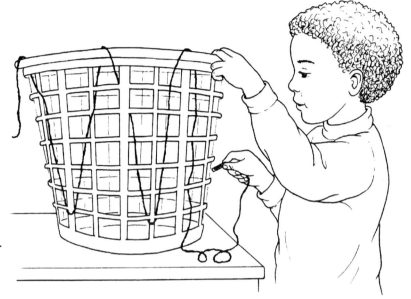

Preparation:

Place a laundry basket right-side-up on a table and tie one end of the yarn to a section of the laundry basket. Create a "long needle" by cutting 1 to 1½ inches of tape and placing it on the other end of the yarn.

1. Demonstrate lacing the yarn through the different holes of the laundry basket, working from side-to-side and up-and-down. Encourage the child to use both hands to push and pull the yarn through the pretend "Swiss cheese."

2. Once the yarn is completely laced through the laundry basket, have the child try to figure out how to unlace the yarn without tangling it. You will most likely need to offer clues such as, "Which hole should we put the yarn in: this one or that one?"

ADAPTATIONS:

To make this activity easier . . .

- If the laundry basket is too cumbersome for your child, weave on paper dinner plates. Prepare the plate by punching holes through it.

- Shorter yarn is easier to manage. Start with a length of yarn that is 12 to 18 inches and increase the length as the child becomes more successful.

To make this activity harder . . .

• Create a design on one side of the laundry basket and ask your child to copy it on the other side of the basket. Eventually, he can practice simple shapes or letters on this surface.

• Turn the laundry basket upside down, making lacing on the inside more difficult.

WHY:

This activity primarily encourages . . .

Bilateral coordination: the ability of the hands to work together as a team. This is essential for complex tasks such as stringing beads or tying shoes.

Eye-hand coordination: the ability of the brain to coordinate information from the eyes with the precise movements of the hand. This is necessary for catching a ball or copying a design from a chalkboard.

Motor planning: the ability to interact with things in the world around you in a purposeful way based on the information perceived through the senses. This means having the idea of what to with something, planning how to do it and then carrying out the plan. This can be seen when a child comes upon an unfamiliar task such as spinning a new top or playing Simon Says.

Separation of two sides of the hand: the use of the thumb and index and middle fingers to push, poke, turn or grasp objects while the pinky side of the hand is supported in the palm. This is essential to correctly grasp a pencil or scissors.

COMMENTS:

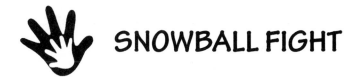 # SNOWBALL FIGHT

MATERIALS:

- newspaper

- scissors

HOW TO:

Preparation:

Cut the newspaper into half sheets. If the child can already cut, he can assist with this task.

1. Have the child take a half sheet of newspaper and crush it into a tight ball. Encourage him to squeeze and shape it with both hands, making sure to emphasize that he "make a tight ball so that the snowball doesn't fall apart." Have him make several snowballs.

2. Position targets around the room and work on tossing the snowballs at them.

3. Clean up the snowballs by having the child crawl on his hands and knees to scoop up the balls and place them in the trash or recycling bin.

ADAPTATIONS:

To make this activity easier . .

- Use a less resistant paper such as tissue.

- Give the child smaller pieces of paper that require less squeezing.

To make this activity harder . . .

- Use a more resistant paper such as magazine paper.

- Give the child a whole sheet of newspaper for more resistance.

- Set up a moving target, such as a large rolling ball or a child running.

- Encourage the child to throw the snowball up into the air and catch it with one or both hands.

WHY:

This activity primarily encourages . . .

Bilateral coordination: the ability of the hands to work together as a team. This is essential for more complex tasks such as stringing beads or tying shoes.

Eye-hand coordination: the ability of the brain to coordinate information from the eyes with the precise movements of the hand. This is necessary for catching a ball or copying a design from a chalkboard.

Release: the letting go of an object by the hand. This is used when putting dishes in the dishwasher or throwing a ball.

Shoulder strength and stability: the ability of the muscles in the shoulders to activate when using the arms. This is used for wheelbarrow walking, carrying heavy boxes or keeping the arms lifted to erase a chalkboard.

COMMENTS:

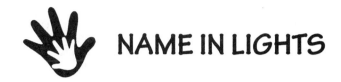

NAME IN LIGHTS

MATERIALS:

- construction paper

- marker and pencil

- carpet square or carpeted area on the floor

- 1 pushpin with a plastic handle

HOW TO:

Preparation:

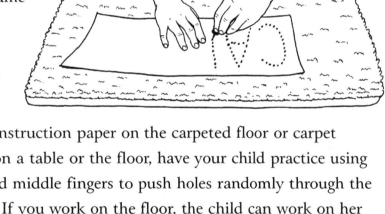

Cut a rectangular shape from construction paper and print your child's first name in pencil. Then use the marker to draw a small dot every 1/4 inch along the letters of her name.

1. Place a scrap piece of construction paper on the carpeted floor or carpet square. Working either on a table or the floor, have your child practice using her thumb and index and middle fingers to push holes randomly through the paper with the pushpin. If you work on the floor, the child can work on her tummy, propped up on her elbows, or sitting with the work between her spread legs.

2. Give your child the piece of construction paper with her preprinted name and ask her to use the pushpin to poke holes where you drew the dots. Encourage her to use one hand to hold the construction paper still and the other hand to control the pushpin. Direct her to poke the dots in a consecutive order, starting at the letter on the left and proceeding to the right, as in reading or writing.

3. When the child has completed her name, she can hold up her pushpin paper in a doorway or window to see her name in lights!

ADAPTATIONS:

To make this activity easier . . .

- Make the dots more noticeable by highlighting them with a brightly colored marker.

- If the child has difficulty pushing through the paper, have her practice by pinning pictures from a magazine on a cork or foam board.

- Teach simple shapes by using the same procedure for creating circles, squares or triangles. Turn the design over to "feel the shape" with your finger by following the bumpy trail created by the pushpin.

To make this activity harder . . .

- Use firm paper such as poster board or used manila folders to create more resistance against the pushpin.

- Place the activity on an easel with a carpet square or foam board behind the paper.

WHY:

This activity primarily encourages . . .

Eye-hand coordination: the ability of the brain to coordinate information from the eyes with the precise movements of the hand. This is necessary for catching a ball or copying a design from a chalkboard.

Handedness: the use of one hand more than the other in one-handed or two-handed activities. This is necessary for skilled tasks like painting a picture or cutting with scissors.

Precision grasp: the ability to use the pads of one's thumb, index finger and, sometimes, middle finger to pick up or manipulate an object, with slight bending of the fingers. This is essential for picking up a raisin or unzipping a small zipper.

206

Separation of two sides of the hand: the use of the thumb and index and middle fingers to push, poke, turn or grasp objects while the pinky side of the hand is supported in the palm. This is essential to correctly grasp a pencil or scissors.

COMMENTS:

NOTE: An adult should supervise small children when provided with small objects or toys. If swallowed, these objects can cause choking, leading to death.

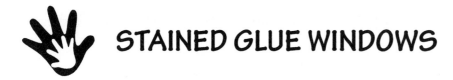 # STAINED GLUE WINDOWS

MATERIALS:

- lid to a small margarine container
- food coloring
- school glue in a small squeeze bottle
- ribbon
- small decorative pieces such as beads, string, tinsel, aluminum foil

HOW TO:

Preparation:

Add food coloring to the glue, stirring or shaking until the color is consistent throughout.

1. Ask the child to pick up the decorative items (beads, foil, etc.) and arrange them in the margarine lid.

2. Demonstrate squeezing the glue bottle. Allow the child to squeeze the glue out of the bottle using both hands, completely filling the lid.

3. Let the lid dry for 24 hours. After it dries, you can peel the glue disk out of the lid and punch a hole through the glue layer using a pen or pencil. This is your stained glue window.

4. The child can then string a ribbon through the hole and tie it off with your help. Hang the decorated disk in a window.

ADAPTATIONS:

To make this activity easier . . .

- Have the child pour the glue into the lid if he is unable to generate the strength for squeezing.

208

- Flatten a ball of play dough and have the child push beads into it to create a design.

To make this activity harder . . .

- Have the child copy a decorative pattern from an already completed stained glue window.

- Have the child squeeze small dots of one color into the lid. Let it dry. Prepare another color of glue and finish filling up the lid with it. Controlled squeezing, such as when making dots, is more difficult than using a full-blown power grasp with constant squeezing.

- Have the child peel the dried glue window out of the lid and poke the hole. Have him lace and tie the string.

WHY:

This activity primarily encourages . . .

Bilateral coordination: the ability of the hands to work together as a team. This is essential for more complex tasks such as stringing beads or tying shoes.

Eye-hand coordination: the ability of the brain to coordinate information from the eyes with the precise movements of the hand. This is necessary for catching a ball or copying a design from a chalkboard.

Motor planning: the ability to interact with things in the world around you in a purposeful way based on the information perceived through the senses. This means having the idea of what to with something, planning how to do it and then carrying out the plan. This can be seen when a child comes upon an unfamiliar task such as spinning a new top or playing Simon Says.

Power grasp: the use of force or power on an object with the fingers and thumb acting against the palm of the hand when grasping that object. This is used when pulling a wagon with something heavy in it or opening a jelly jar.

(continued)

COMMENTS:

NOTE: An adult should supervise small children when provided with small objects or toys. If swallowed, these objects can cause choking, leading to death.

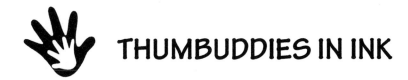

THUMBUDDIES IN INK

MATERIALS:

- nontoxic inkpads
- paper
- markers

HOW TO:

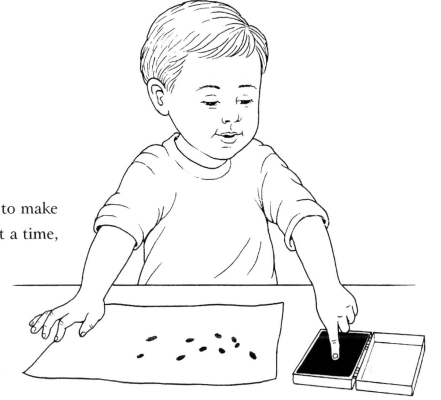

1. Demonstrate how to make fingerprints, one at a time, by straightening each finger and pressing the pad into the inkpad and then onto the paper.

2. Encourage the child to use all his fingers to decorate his paper with fingerprints.

3. Invite the child to use a marker to attach arms and legs to each fingerprint. If the child has difficulty filling in the detail, encourage him to look into a mirror and draw on the fingerprints all of the facial features he sees on himself.

ADAPTATIONS:

To make this activity easier . . .

- Have the child make the fingerprints and you add the facial features.
- Have the child use only his index finger and thumb to make the fingerprints.
- Have the child make handprints on the paper.

Handprints–Pieraccini and Vance

To make this activity harder . . .

- Tape the paper to the wall.

- Provide the child with a variety of stamping tools such as stamping blocks and rollers or sponges to encourage different types of grasps and movements.

- Have the child tell a story using each finger as a different character. On several recipe cards, have him illustrate the story making a different fingerprint for each character. You can write the text to the story and use tape to bind the cards together into a book.

- Have the child imitate a color sequence, such as one purple fingerprint and two green fingerprints in a row.

WHY:

This activity primarily encourages . . .

Eye-hand coordination: the ability of the brain to coordinate information from the eyes with the precise movements of the hand. This is necessary for catching a ball or copying a design from a chalkboard.

Isolated finger movements: the ability to move the fingers independently, whether fingers are being used individually or in combination with each other. This is necessary to rotate the dial on a pop-up toy or snap fingers to music.

Separation of two sides of the hand: the use of the thumb and index and middle fingers to push, poke, turn or grasp objects while the pinky side of the hand is supported in the palm of the hand. This is essential to correctly grasp a pencil or scissors.

Visual Perception: the ability to perceive and understand information received from the eyes. This is used when playing follow-the-leader or distinguishing the difference between the letters "d" and "b" when reading.

COMMENTS:

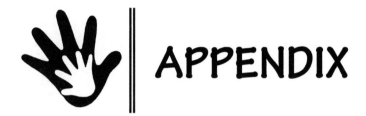

APPENDIX

Which Activity, Which Hand Skills?

Instructions

The chart on the next two pages will help you choose an appropriate activity for your client's area of need. First locate the identified hand skill in the left-hand or right-hand column. Then locate all the activities that incorporate that skill by looking for the squares with Xs in the column next to that skill. Then follow those columns up to the the activity title.

Which Activity, Which Hand Skills?

	Ball Games (p.151)	Beans and Rice (p.133)	Confetti Makers (p.153)	Creepy Crawly (p.136)	Dippity Do® Writing (p.185)	Edible Jewelry (p.187)	Feeding Our Furry Friends (p.192)	Feely Box (p.138)	Golf Ball Roll (p.156)	Goop (p.159)	Green Thumb (p.162)	Hats Off (p.141)	Juice Makers (p.190)	Lacing Through Swiss Cheese (p.201)	Mirror, Mirror on the Wall (p.143)
Bilateral Coordination	X	X	X	X	X	X			X	X	X	X	X	X	X
Eye-Hand Coordination	X	X	X		X	X	X		X		X	X		X	X
Fine Motor Skills	X	X	X	X	X	X	X	X	X	X	X	X	X	X	X
Forearm Pronation and Supination	X	X							X	X	X	X		X	
Handedness	X		X		X	X	X		X		X			X	X
Haptic Sense		X			X			X		X	X		X		
In-Hand Manipulation						X		X		X				X	
Isolated Finger Movement		X			X					X	X				
Motor Planning				X	X	X	X		X	X	X	X		X	X
Power Grasp	X	X							X	X	X	X	X		
Precision Grasp		X	X			X			X	X			X		
Reach	X	X	X	X	X	X	X	X		X	X	X	X	X	X
Release	X		X			X	X	X		X	X	X		X	
Separation of Two Sides of the Hand		X	X	X	X	X	X				X			X	
Shoulder Strength and Stability	X			X	X		X		X	X	X	X	X	X	X
Trunk Stability	X			X					X		X			X	X
Visual Perception		X			X	X	X		X			X		X	X

Which Activity, Which Hand Skills?

Musical Pots (p. 145)	Name in Lights (p. 205)	Paint Your World with Water (p. 165)	Pizza Dough (p. 168)	Polka Dot Flowers (p. 198)	Potato Porcupine (p. 171)	Putting Money in the Bank (p. 173)	Snowball Fight (p. 203)	Sponges and Buckets (p. 176)	Stained Glue Windows (p. 208)	Sticky Ball (p. 147)	String Art (p. 178)	Tear-It-Up Designs (p. 181)	Thumbuddies in Ink (p. 211)	Window Washers (p. 195)	
X	X	X	X		X	X	X	X	X	X		X		X	Bilateral Coordination
X	X	X	X	X	X	X	X	X	X	X	X	X	X		Eye-Hand Coordination
X	X	X	X	X	X	X	X	X	X	X	X	X	X	X	Fine Motor Skills
X		X			X			X		X		X		X	Forearm Pronation and Supination
	X	X	X	X	X	X	X		X		X		X	X	Handedness
		X					X	X		X					Haptic Sense
		X		X	X				X						In-Hand Manipulation
		X										X			Isolated Finger Movement
	X	X	X	X	X	X		X	X		X	X			Motor Planning
X	X	X		X	X		X	X	X	X		X		X	Power Grasp
	X		X	X	X	X			X		X	X			Precision Grasp
X	X	X	X	X	X	X	X	X	X	X	X	X	X	X	Reach
		X	X	X	X	X	X	X			X	X			Release
	X		X	X	X	X			X		X	X	X		Separation of Two Sides of the Hand
X		X			X	X	X	X	X		X	X		X	Shoulder Strength and Stability
X		X					X	X	X	X				X	Trunk Stability
	X	X		X		X	X		X						Visual Perception

Which Activity, Which Hand Skills in Daily Activities?

The chart below will help you choose an appropriate activity for your client's area of need. First locate the specific hand skill in daily activities in the left-hand or right-hand column. Then locate all the activities that incorporate that skill by looking for the squares with Xs in them. Then follow those columns up to the the activity title.

	Ball Games (p. 151)	Beans and Rice (p. 133)	Confetti Makers (p. 153)	Creepy Crawly (p. 136)	Dippity Do® Writing (p. 185)	Edible Jewelry (p. 187)	Feeding Our Furry Friends (p. 192)	Feely Box (p. 138)	Golf Ball Roll (p. 156)	Goop (p. 159)	Green Thumb (p. 162)	Hats Off (p. 141)	Juice Makers (p. 190)	Lacing Through Swiss Cheese (p. 201)	Mirror, Mirror, on the Wall (p. 143)
Hand Skills in Ball Play	X														
Hand Skills in Coloring				X											
Hand Skills in Dressing					X							X		X	
Hand Skills in Drinking													X		
Hand Skills in Feeding						X	X		X						
Hand Skills in Play	X	X	X	X	X	X	X	X	X	X	X	X	X	X	
Hand Skills in Printing				X											
Hand Skills in Scissors Use		X				X									
Hand Skills in Sign Language															X
Hand Skills in Tool Use		X	X				X		X	X					

Which Activity, Which Hand Skills in Daily Activities?

Musical Pots (p. 145)	Name in Lights (p. 205)	Paint Your World with Water (p. 165)	Pizza Dough (p. 168)	Polka Dot Flowers (p. 198)	Potato Porcupine (p. 171)	Putting Money in the Bank (p. 173)	Snowball Fight (p. 203)	Sponges and Buckets (p. 176)	Stained Glue Windows (p. 208)	Sticky Ball (p. 147)	String Art (p. 178)	Tear-It-Up Designs (p. 181)	Thumbuddies in Ink (p. 211)	Window Washers (p. 195)	
							X								Hand Skills in Ball Play
		X											X		Hand Skills in Coloring
						X									Hand Skills in Dressing
															Hand Skills in Drinking
															Hand Skills in Feeding
X	X	X	X	X	X	X	X	X	X	X	X	X	X	X	Hand Skills in Play
	X												X		Hand Skills in Printing
															Hand Skills in Scissors Use
															Hand Skills in Sign Language
	X	X		X		X						X		X	Hand Skills in Tool Use

Activity Checklist

To track when articles and activities were provided to your client's care-giver, record the dates in the area provided next to each handout.

Child's Name:

DOB:

Parent/Caregiver's Name:

Hand Skills and Related Topics Articles

	Date										
Hand Structure											
Fine Motor Skills											
Bilateral Coordination											
Release											
Upper Extremity Weightbearing											
Shoulder Strength and Stability											
Reach											
Precision Grasp											
Trunk Stability											
Eye-Hand Coordination											
Isolated Finger Movement											
Separation of Two Sides of the Hand											
In-Hand Manipulation											
Forearm Pronation and Supination											
Handedness											
Power Grasp											
Motor Planning											
Visual Perception											
Haptic Sense											

Daily Activities Articles

	Date										
Hand Skills in Sign Language											
Hand Skills in Drinking											
Hand Skills in Feeding											
Hand Skills in Dressing											
Hand Skills in Play											
Hand Skills in Tool Use											
Hand Skills in Ball Play											
Hand Skills in Coloring											
Hand Skills in Scissors Use											
Hand Skills in Printing											

Adaptations Articles

Incorporating Activities into the Day											
One-Hand Adaptations											
Activity Preparation and Position											
Environmental Adaptations											
Positioning the Child											
Presentation of Task											
The Just Right Challenge											
Properties of Toys											
Use of the Vertical Plane											
Adaptations for Left-Handedness											
Pre-writing Adaptations											

Activities

	Date										
Beans and Rice											
Creepy Crawly											
Feely Box											
Hats Off											
Mirror, Mirror, on the Wall											
Musical Pots											
Sticky Ball											
Ball Games											
Confetti Makers											
Golf Ball Roll											
Goop											
Green Thumb											
Paint Your World with Water											
Pizza Dough											
Potato Porcupine											
Putting Money in the Bank											
Sponges and Buckets											
String Art											
Tear-It-Up Designs											
Dippity Do® Writing											
Edible Jewelry											
Juice Makers											
Feeding Our Furry Friends											
Window Washers											
Polka Dot Flowers											
Lacing Through Swiss Cheese											
Snowball Fight											
Name in Lights											
Stained Glue Windows											
Thumbuddies in Ink											

Toys, Toys and More Toys

Is a birthday or holiday coming up? Or do you want to buy a toy that will challenge your child? The following list suggests toys in different developmental age categories and includes the two primary hand skills each toy promotes. The age category represents when the toy will first provide a challenge for the child while still allowing for success. Many of the toys, like the easel, are appropriate past the age for which they are first mentioned.

3 Months to 1 Year

Toy:	Skills:
soft blocks	reach, grasp
rattle	reach, grasp
mobile	reach, visual-perceptual skills
infant mirror	reach, visual-perceptual skills
busy box	reach, shoulder strength and stability
activity gym	reach, shoulder strength and stability
playmat	haptic sense, shoulder strength and stability
pull toy	grasp, shoulder strength and stability
soft ball	grasp, eye-hand coordination
bubbles	reach, eye-hand coordination
soft ring stacker	grasp, eye-hand coordination
textured book	grasp, haptic sense

Toys, Toys and More Toys

1 to 2 Years

Toy:	Skills:
1" beads and stiff string	precision grasp, bilateral coordination
form board with 3 geometric shapes	visual-perceptual skills, eye-hand coordination
shape sorter	visual-perceptual skills, eye-hand coordination
cardboard book	precision grasp, bilateral coordination
bead maze on wires	eye-hand coordination, forearm supination and pronation
pop-up toy	precision grasp, isolated finger movements
hammer toy	power grasp, eye-hand coordination
Koosh® Ball	power grasp, haptic sense
beach ball	eye-hand coordination, bilateral coordination
See 'n Say®	power grasp, bilateral coordination
musical book	precision grasp, isolated finger movements
push-button play phone	isolated finger movements, bilateral coordination
shovel and bucket	power grasp, forearm pronation and supination

Toys, Toys and More Toys

2 to 3 Years

Toy:	Skills:
1" beads and string	precision grasp, bilateral coordination
bank and coins	precision grasp, bilateral coordination
paper book	in-hand manipulation, bilateral coordination
jack-in-the-box	precision grasp, shoulder strength and stability
nesting cups	eye-hand coordination, shoulder strength and stability
Easter eggs filled with small toys	precision grasp, bilateral coordination
form board with pegs on pieces	precision grasp, visual-perceptual skills
Magna Doodle® and design stampers	precision grasp, eye-hand coordination
preschool crayons	precision grasp, eye-hand coordination
child's figure markers	precision grasp, eye-hand coordination
Colorforms®	precision grasp, eye-hand coordination
flannel boards and figures	precision grasp, eye-hand coordination
stamps	precision grasp, eye-hand coordination
sponge stencils	precision grasp, eye-hand coordination
magnetic letters and shapes	precision grasp, eye-hand coordination
pop beads	power grasp, bilateral coordination
easy-grip pegs and pegboard	precision grasp, shoulder strength and stability
large Lego® blocks (Duplo®)	power grasp, eye-hand coordination
Play Doh®	power grasp, bilateral coordination
tea and kitchen set	precision grasp, forearm supination and pronation
sliceable fruit and vegetables	power grasp, bilateral coordination
xylophone	power grasp, eye-hand coordination
easel	reach, shoulder strength and stability
chalkboard and chalk	reach, shoulder strength and stability
dry erase board and markers	reach, shoulder strength and stability
crawling tunnel	trunk stability, shoulder strength and stability

Toys, Toys and More Toys

3 to 4 Years

Toy:	Skills:
hand puppets	separation of two sides of hand, isolated finger movements
standard crayons	precision grasp, eye-hand coordination
standard markers	precision grasp, eye-hand coordination
sidewalk chalk	precision grasp, eye-hand coordination
roller stamps	precision grasp, eye-hand coordination
watercolor brushes	precision grasp, eye-hand coordination
Magna Doodle® and magnetic pen	precision grasp, eye-hand coordination
child's scissors	precision grasp, separation of two sides of hand
construction blocks	precision grasp, motor planning
bristle blocks	power grasp, motor planning
dressing doll with fasteners	precision grasp, bilateral coordination
child's cash register with coins	isolated finger movements, in-hand manipulation
counting abacus	isolated finger movements, precision grasp
interlocking puzzle with 10 or fewer pieces	precision grasp, visual-perceptual skills
child's nuts and bolts	precision grasp, in-hand manipulation
Silly Putty®	power grasp, bilateral coordination
drum with drumsticks	precision grasp, bilateral coordination
rainmaker	forearm pronation and supination, shoulder strength and stability
cymbals	bilateral coordination, shoulder strength and stability
magnetic wand	power grasp, eye-hand coordination
fishing game	eye-hand coordination, shoulder strength and stability
beginners' basketball hoop	release, eye-hand coordination

Toys, Toys and More Toys

4 to 5 Years

Toy:	Skills:
lacing shapes	precision grasp, eye-hand coordination
Tinker Toys®	motor planning, eye-hand coordination
pick-up sticks	precision grasp, visual-perceptual skills
marbles and jacks	bilateral coordination, eye-hand coordination
constructional marble runs	precision grasp, motor planning
Slinky®	power grasp, bilateral coordination
Etch A Sketch®	precision grasp, eye-hand coordination
interlocking puzzle with 10 or more pieces	precision grasp, visual-perceptual skills
Cootie®	precision grasp, eye-hand coordination
Bed Bugs®	precision grasp, eye-hand coordination
Lincoln Logs®	motor planning, eye-hand coordination
remote-control cars	isolated finger movement, eye-hand coordination
croquet	bilateral coordination, eye-hand coordination
horse shoes	release, eye-hand coordination
child's bowling set	release, eye-hand coordination
T-ball set	bilateral coordination, eye-hand coordination
Velcro® catching mitt with ball	release, eye-hand coordination
jump rope	power grasp, bilateral coordination

GLOSSARY

Glossary

Bilateral coordination: the ability of the hands to work together as a team. This is essential for more complex tasks such as stringing beads or tying shoes.

Eye-hand coordination: the ability of the brain to coordinate information from the eyes with the precise movements of the hand. This is necessary for catching a ball or copying a design from a chalkboard.

Forearm pronation and supination: the ability to move the forearm back and forth between the positions of palm facing down and palm facing up. This is used when scooping food from a plate or giving a "high-5" to a friend.

Handedness: the use of one hand more than the other in one-handed or two-handed activities. This is necessary for skilled tasks like painting a picture or cutting with scissors.

Haptic sense: the ability to gather information about or identify objects only through touch when manipulating them with the hands. This is used when reaching in a backpack for an eraser or buttoning a shirt under your chin without looking.

In-hand manipulation: the ability of the fingers and palm to turn, twist and move an object in the hand. This is important for opening a screw-top container, turning a coin between the fingertips or writing with a pencil.

Isolated finger movements: the ability to move the fingers independently of each other, whether fingers are being used individually or in combination with each other. This is necessary to rotate the dial on a pop-up toy or snap fingers to music.

Motor planning: the ability to interact with things in the world around you in a purposeful way based on the information perceived through the senses. This means having the idea of what to with something, planning how to do it and then carrying out the plan. This can be seen when a child comes upon an unfamiliar task such as spinning a new top or playing Simon Says.

Power grasp: the use of force or power on an object with the fingers and thumb acting against the palm of the hand when grasping that object. This is used when pulling a wagon with something heavy in it or opening a jelly jar.

Precision grasp: the ability to use the pads of your thumb, index finger and, sometimes, middle finger to pick up or manipulate an object, with slight bending of the fingers. This is essential for picking up a raisin or unzipping a small zipper.

Reach: the ability to extend the arm to obtain, release or hold an object. This is used when getting a toy from a shelf or catching a ball.

Release: the letting go of an object by the hand. This is used when putting dishes in the dishwasher or throwing a ball.

Separation of two sides of the hand: the use of the thumb and index and middle fingers to push, poke, turn or grasp objects while the pinky side of the hand is supported in the palm. This is essential to correctly grasp a pencil or scissors.

Shoulder strength and stability: the ability of the muscles in the shoulders to activate when using the arms. This is used for wheelbarrow walking, carrying heavy boxes or keeping your arms lifted to erase a chalkboard.

Trunk stability: the stability in the body's trunk to maintain an upright posture, shift weight in all directions and rotate the trunk to the left and right. This is necessary for sitting on a bench while doing a puzzle or leaning forward to pick up a toy.

Visual Perception: the ability to perceive and understand information received from the eyes. This is used when playing follow-the-leader or distinguishing the difference between the letters "d" and "b" when reading.

REFERENCES

References

Acredolo, L., and Goodwyn, S. *Baby Signs: How to Talk with Your Baby Before Your Baby Can Talk.* Chicago: Contemporary Books, 1996.

Alexander, R., Boehme, R., and Cupps, B. *Normal Development of Functional Motor Skills: The First Year of Life.* Tucson, AZ: Therapy Skill Builders, 1993.

Alston, J., and Taylor, J. *Handwriting: Theory, Research and Practice.* New York: Nichols Publishing Company, 1987.

Ayres, A. J. *Developmental Dyspraxia and Adult-Onset Apraxia.* Torrance CA: Sensory Integration International, 1985.

Ballinger, B. Visual influences in the learning process. *Sensory Integration Quarterly,* vol. 22, no. 1: 1-4 (1995).

Bartlett, D. J., and Palisano, R. J. A multivariate model of determinants of motor change for children with cerebral palsy. *Journal of Physical Therapy,* vol. 80, no. 6: 598-611 (2000).

Benbow, M. Principles and practices of teaching handwriting. In A. Henderson and C. Pehoski (Eds.), *Hand Function in the Child: Foundations for Remediation.* St. Louis, MO: Mosby Year Book, 1995.

Boehme, R. Developing hand function. In B. M. Connolly and P. C. Montgomery (Eds.), *Therapeutic Exercise in Developmental Disabilities* (2nd ed.). Hixson, TN: Chattanooga Group, 1993.

Burton, A. W., and Dancisak, M. J. Grip form and graphomotor control in preschool children. *American Journal of Occupational Therapy,* vol. 54, no. 1: 10-17 (2000).

Case-Smith, J. Grasp, release, and bimanual skills in the first two years of life. In A. Henderson and C. Pehoski (Eds.), *Hand Function in the Child: Foundations for Remediation.* St. Louis, MO: Mosby Year Book, 1995.

Cunningham Amundson, S. J. Handwriting: Evaluation and intervention in school settings. In J. Case-Smith and C. Pehoski (Eds.), *Development of Hand Skills in the Child.* Bethesda, MD: American Occupational Therapy Association, Inc., 1992.

Duff, S. V. Prehension. In D. Cech, and S.T. Martin (Eds.) *Functional Movement Development Across the Life Span.* Philadelphia, PA: W. B. Saunders Company, 1995.

Dunn, M. *Pre-Dressing Skills.* Tucson, AZ: Communication Skill Builders, 1983. (Now available from Austin, TX: Pro Ed.)

Dunn, M. *Pre-Sign Language Motor Skills.* Tucson, AZ: Communication Skill Builders, 1982.

Effgen, S. K. Developing postural control. In B. M. Connolly and P. C. Montgomery (Eds.), *Therapeutic Exercise in Developmental Disabilities* (2nd ed.). Hixson, TN: Chattanooga Group, 1993.

Eisenberg, A., Murkoff, H. E., and Hathaway, S. E. *What to Expect: The Toddler Years.* New York: Workman Publishing Company Inc., 1994.

Erhardt, R. P. *Developmental Hand Dysfunction: Theory, Assessment and Treatment* (2nd ed.). Tucson, AZ: Therapy Skill Builders, 1994.

Erhardt, R. P. Eye-hand coordination. In J. Case-Smith and C. Pehoski, (Eds.), *Development of Hand Skills in the Child.* Bethesda, MD: American Occupational Therapy Association, Inc., 1992.

Erhardt, R. P. The transition from finger feeding to utensil use: A systems approach. *Advance for Occupational Therapy Practitioners,* vol. 15, no. 22: 23-25 (1999).

Exner, C. E. Development of hand skills. In J. Case-Smith, A. S. Allen, and P. N. Pratt (Eds.), *Occupational Therapy for Children.* (3rd ed). St. Louis, MO: Mosby, 1996.

Exner, C. E. In-hand manipulation skills. In J. Case-Smith and C. Pehoski (Eds.), *Development of Hand Skills in the Child.* Bethesda, MD: American Occupational Therapy Association, 1992.

Exner, C .E. Remediation of hand skill problems in children. In A. Henderson and C. Pehoski (Eds.), *Hand Function in the Child: Foundations for Remediation.* St. Louis, MO: Mosby Year Book, 1995.

Fisher, A. G., Murray, E. A., and Bundy, A. C. *Sensory Integration: Theory and Practice.* Philadelphia, PA: F.A. Davis Company, 1991.

Folio, M. and Fewell, R. *Peabody Developmental Motor Scales.* Allen, TX: DLM Teaching Resources, 1983.

Henderson, A. Self-care and hand skill. In A. Henderson and C. Pehoski (Eds.), *Hand Function in the Child: Foundations for Remediation.* St. Louis, MO: Mosby Year Book, 1995.

234

Higgins, S. Motor skill acquisition. *Journal of Physical Therapy,* vol. 71, no. 2: 123-139 (1991).

Humphries, T., Padden, C., and O'Rourke, T. *A Basic Course In American Sign Language* (2nd ed.). Silver Springs, MD: T. J. Publishers Inc., 1994.

Johnson-Martin, N., Attermeier, S. M., and Hacker, B. *Carolina Curriculum for Preschoolers with Special Needs.* Baltimore, MD: Paul H. Brooks Publishing Company, 1990.

Kamakura, N., Matsuo, M., Harumi, I., Mitsuboshi, F., and Miura, Y. Patterns of static prehension in normal hands. *American Journal of Occupational Therapy,* vol. 34, no. 7: 437-445 (1980).

Link, L., Lukens, S., and Bush, M. A. Spherical grip strength in children 3 to 6 years of age. *American Journal of Occupational Therapy,* vol. 49, no. 4: 318-325 (1995).

Malick, M. H., and Meyer Dip, C. M. H. *Manual on Management of the Quadriplegic Upper Extremity.* Pittsburgh, PA: Maude H. Malick, 1978.

Marmer, L. Climbing to maturity hand over hand. *Advance for Occupational Therapists,* vol. 13, no. 20: 13 and 19 (1997).

Miller, K. *Things to Do with Toddlers and Twos* (4th ed.). Telshare Publishing, 1984.

Murray, E. Hand preference and its development. In A. Henderson and C. Pehoski (Eds.), *Hand Function in the Child: Foundations for Remediation.* St. Louis, MO: Mosby Year Book, 1995.

Myers, C. M. Therapeutic fine-motor activities for preschoolers. In J. Case-Smith and C. Pehoski (Eds.), *Development of Hand Skills in the Child.* Bethesda, MD: American Occupational Therapy Association, Inc., 1992.

Olsen, J. Z. *Handwriting without Tears.* Potomac, MD: Janice Z. Olsen, 1997.

Olsen, J. Z. *Printing: Teacher's Guide.* Potomac, MD: Janice Z. Olsen, 1997.

Punwar, A. *Occupational Therapy: Principles and Practice.* Baltimore, MD: Williams and Wilkins, 1988.

Reed, K., and Sanderson, S., *Concepts of Occupational Therapy* (2nd ed.). Baltimore, MD: Williams and Wilkins, 1983.

Reeves, G. D. Influence of somatic activity on body scheme. *Sensory Integration Quarterly,* vol. 8, no. 2: 1-2 (1985).

Rosblad, B. Reaching and eye-hand coordination. In A. Henderson and C. Pehoski (Eds.), *Hand Function in the Child: Foundations for Remediation.* St. Louis, MO: Mosby Year Book, 1995.

Schaaf, R.C. Play behavior and occupational therapy. *American Journal of Occupational Therapy,* vol. 44, no. 10: 68-75 (1990).

Schneck, C., and Battaglia, C. Developing scissors skills in young children. In J. Case-Smith, and C. Pehoski (Eds.), *Development of Hand Skills in the Child.* Bethesda, MD: American Occupational Therapy Association, 1992.

Schneck, C., and Henderson, A. Descriptive analysis of the developmental progression of grip position for pencil and crayon control in non-dysfunctional children. *American Journal of Occupational Therapy,* vol. 44, no. 10: 893-900 (1990).

Stahl, C. Developing the skills for refined sign-language expression. *Advance for Occupational Therapists,* vol. 13, no. 20: 14-15 (1997).

Stilwell, J. M., and Cermack, S.A. Perceptual functions of the hand. In A. Henderson and C. Pehoski (Eds.), *Hand Function in the Child: Foundations for Remediation.* St. Louis, MO: Mosby Year Book, 1995.

Strickland, J. Anatomy and kinesiology of the hand. In A. Henderson and C. Pehoski (Eds.), *Hand Function in the Child: Foundations for Remediation.* St. Louis, MO: Mosby Year Book, 1995.

Tseng, M. H., and Cermack, S. A. The influence of ergonomic factors and perceptual-motor abilities on handwriting performance. *American Journal of Occupational Therapy,* vol. 47, no. 10: 919-926 (1993).

Vergara, E. R. Typical and atypical development of feeding. In *Foundations for Practice in the Neonatal Intensive Care and Early Intervention: A Self-Guided Practice Manual,* vol. 2. Rockville, MD: American Occupational Therapy Association, 1993.

Vergara, E. R. Typical and atypical fine-motor development. In *Foundations for Practice in the Neonatal Intensive Care and Early Intervention: A Self-Guided Practice Manual,* vol. 2. Rockville, MD: The American Occupational Therapy Association, 1993.

Weil, M . J., and Cunningham Amundson, S. J. Relationship between visuomotor and handwriting skills of children in kindergarten. *American Journal of Occupational Therapy,* vol. 48, no. 11: 982-988 (1994).

White, D. Signing instead of whining. *The Commercial Appeal,* July 18, 1999: G1, G4. Memphis, TN: Memphis Publishing Co.

Windsor, M. Clinical interpretation of "grip form and graphomotor control in pre-school children." *American Journal of Occupational Therapy,* vol. 54, no. 1: 18-19 (2000).

Ziviani, J. Pencil grasp and manipulation. In J. Alston and J. Taylor (Eds.), *Handwriting: Theory, Research and Practice.* New York: Nichols Publishing Company, 1987.

Ziviani, J. The development of graphomotor skills. In A. Henderson and C. Pehoski (Eds.), *Hand Function in the Child: Foundations for Remediation.* St. Louis, MO: Mosby Year Book, 1995.

About the Authors

Valerie Pieraccini graduated from Western Michigan University in Kalamazoo, Michigan, with a bachelor's degree in occupational therapy in 1988. She has worked in pediatrics for most of her career. She obtained her certificate to administer the Sensory Integration Praxis Test in 1995. Valerie lives in Phoenix, Arizona. Her greatest enjoyment is raising her sons, Lucas and Alex, with her husband, Paul. She also enjoys long walks, gardening and traveling.

Darla Vance graduated from DePauw University in Greencastle, Indiana, with a bachelor's degree in psychology in 1988 and from Western Michigan University in Kalamazoo, Michigan, with a master's degree in occupational therapy in 1990. Darla has been active in the pediatric field in a variety of settings and has been a speaker at national conventions presenting on sensory integration issues. She presently resides in Phoenix, Arizona. Darla enjoys hiking in the desert, yoga, running, playing the guitar and hanging out with her family and her animals.

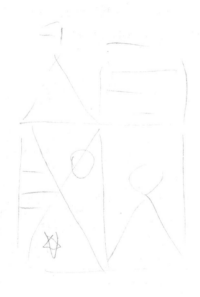